So Close to

Death

Yet So Far

Away

By Derek C. Evans

This book is dedicated to all those out there suffering from Dysautonomia and Postural Orthostatic Tachycardia Syndrome (P.O.T.S.). As well as all my family, friends and those nearest and dearest to my heart who have stuck with me every step of the way.

Contents

Introduction

Have you ever walked around day after day, month after month, year after year, keeping a secret deep inside you that you were hiding from the whole world? A secret that stuck with you every day of your life, everywhere you went? A secret no one else knew, for the rare exception of a close few? One you never told anyone? You never told anyone because you were afraid. You were afraid they would never believe you. You were afraid they would start to look at you different? Afraid they would no longer view you the same. Scared they would end up judging you. Paranoid that if you did indeed tell someone, the word would get out. And everyone knows how quick rumors can spread and how the truth can get twisted around the more people pass on the story. If the secret were to get out, everyone and their mother would start questioning you about it. It would start to unravel like a domino effect. You don't have the time nor want to deal with the storm that could unleash. So instead of opening up and being honest about your secret, you constantly kept making up excuses to cover up for it. You make up excuses so people would not bother you, hoping they never find out the truth. No matter how stupid your excuse may have seemed, you did it anyway. For whatever reason it never felt like a good idea to reveal the real reason for what had just transpired.

This secret is so influential to the person you were and has had such a tremendous impact on your life. Yet incredibly at the end of the day it never seemed worth it to tell anybody. Deep down your gut told you it was just better to keep it unknown from the rest of the world.

Years go by and it does not seem like a big deal. Everything seems to be going just fine, despite this deep burden you continue to carry with you all the time. You are getting promoted at your job. You are a young adult just starting your career. You get to travel the world with your best friends. Your life can not seem to be going in any better direction. Everything seems positive and on the upswing. It gets to the point you forget you are even carrying this gigantic secret around inside you. It seems as if it is in the distant past. You no longer worry about it. It never dawns on you that at any moment it can creep right up and take everything from you in an instant.

This is exactly how deep secrets are. When you least expect it, they come out of nowhere and stab you in the back. It becomes a sharp pain that hurts you physically, mentally, and emotionally. Dark secret or not, it is almost like karma for never telling anyone about it. Once this happens you are in panic mode. You just had a moment and you are not sure how to explain it. Your job, relationships, and well-being are all on the line. You keep thinking and analyzing what excuse you can create this time to keep moving on. You try to think of another justification to keep your secret hidden. You try to think of another excuse to try and put the secret in the past again, hoping in time it will be in the past for good and never come back.

After the dust settles and you just made up more excuses for the humiliation that had just happened to you, you start to question yourself. Is it really worth keeping the truth a secret anymore? You start to feel different than you used to feel about keeping this secret from everyone now. The difference now is that you are starting to have a change of heart. After almost a decade of hiding this secret from everyone, you feel the urge to open up. The world needs to know. The secret is burning deep inside you. It is beginning to cause more stress, taking its toll on you mentally and physically. The obsession to keep it a secret after so many years is making you feel exhausted.

A decade later you became an adult. At the point in your life where you do not care what anyone thinks. If people judge you so be it. Your skin has grown thicker. You can handle this now. You just want this deep burden off your chest.

This is it. You are dead set on opening up and telling everyone the secret that has haunted you for ten years. The question now is how are you going to tell it? It has been so many years, how are you going to explain it to your job, family, and friends? What is the right way to approach this? When is the right time? Should it be done via social media? Would it be better to tell everyone face to face? Should you start calling people up on the phone? How do you tell the secret you have hidden from the world for a decade? A secret that is so important for people to know yet is going to be so complicated to understand. How can you break it down for them, in the simplest terms so that they can comprehend it? What is the best way? How? Like just how can you pull this off? These are the questions that keep going through your mind over and over.

That question is hard to answer but is one I had to answer myself. For almost decade I held a secret from most of my friends. I held it from high school and college friends. I held it from family members, my job, my co-workers, and the every day to day people I interacted with. I was just like the person I described above. I did not want anyone to know. So to all of my friends that I often made excuses on why I could not hang out at certain times, this is the reason why. For all the times when playing sports, I would become so out of breath and you all did not understand why, this is reason why. All the times it seemed like I was having an anxiety attack or acting as if I was on drugs, this is reason why. Every time I looked horrible and I told you I was fine, though you knew I was lying, this is the reason why. Why it always seemed like I made an excuse for why I could not do something, this is the reason why. Why I decided to write this book, this is the reason why.

The reason is because at seventeen-years-old I was diagnosed with Postural Orthostatic Tachycardia Syndrome, also known as P.O.T.S. Only discovered in 1993, it is a very bizarre syndrome. It is a syndrome that has yet to find a cause or a cure. It is a dysautonomia disorder, an imbalance in the nervous system, with similarities to an autoimmune and many other diseases combined. It is a syndrome usually only determined by a tilt table test. A syndrome that has already affected 1,000,000 people yet is so little known. P.O.T.S. can make a patient look perfectly fine on the outside but yet that same person is so crippled on the inside. This is why it is also known as an "Invisible illness". Postural Orthostatic Tachycardia Syndrome is a disorder so perplexing and so hard to grasp for the average person. Hence, the reason why I kept it a secret for so long.

As you read this book you will start to learn more about this inexplicable syndrome called Postural Orthostatic Tachycardia Syndrome, also known as P.O.T.S. You will learn about the struggles I had to go through, which have so many others with the same disorder. You will hear their stories as well. You will hear stories from doctors and many loved ones that know someone with P.O.T.S. You will see the importance and need to bring awareness to this syndrome. You will begin to realize why after almost a decade I finally decided to come clean about this. The time is now. I want to be honest with everyone about what has really been going on with me the past decade. I decided how I will let everyone know. My answer was to write this book.

The Day that Changed my Life Forever

Did you ever have a day in your life that you look back and reflect on it so much it almost becomes an obsession? You drift back and constantly evaluate everything that happened and consistently wonder what caused the situation at hand. Contemplating what you could have done differently. Yet no matter how much you look back, you realize there is nothing you could have changed. The only thing you can think is how different your life would be if this day would have just never occurred.

In the recent weeks, months and in some cases years after this significant day occurs, you mirror back on it. The memories often fill you with sadness, then anger, sadness and then anger. It is like a repeating cycle. You do not understand why this had to happen to you. What makes you so different from everyone else? Why were you the one chosen? Why were you dealt these cards? As time goes on the sadness and anger fades away. You begin to face the true reality your life will never be the same as it once was. You learn to find happiness again but every so often you drift back and relive this day. As you remember this day, the emotion you feel is not as strong as it once had been. It is slowly just becoming a numb feeling. All you can think about is the same damn question. What if? What if this never happened? Then you start daydreaming for a while picturing all the great things that would have happened had this day never existed. You fantasize how everything would be so much better as if all your goals and dreams would have come true if this day had just never came to fruition.

You snap out of daydream land and come back to reality. You're numb, not really sure how to feel. You accept what has happened even though you do not want to.

Years have passed and you still cannot comprehend everything. Finally, after a brief moment, you realize no need to waste time dwelling on the past and go back on with living your life the best you possibly can no matter how more difficult it has become. You just put a smile on and chug along even though you always remain somewhat confused.

June 16th, 2008. I remember this day perfectly. It was a beautiful sunny day. Not too hot but not too cool. It was a perfect mid 80 degree day in Reading, Pennsylvania. More importantly it was a perfect day to be a lifeguard, which was my summer job at the time. Being seventeen-years-old and involved in sports year around, summers were the only time I could work and make money to help save for college. Working as a lifeguard was the perfect job for me.

As I approached work I was feeling great. Recently, I had started a new weightlifting and vertical exercise program. I was utilizing this program to help increase my athletic ability for all the sports I would be participating in my senior year. Plus, I liked the results I was seeing on my body from working out. Let's be honest. What seventeen-year -old male does not want to look good to impress his fellow high school classmates?

I was a very hard worker, especially when it came to sports. Sports were my life. My life in all seriousness literally revolved around sports. Some of my coaches used to refer to me as a "Warrior", "The energizer bunny" and my fellow teammates would often describe me as someone who has a "Killer instinct". Needless to say, I never lacked motivation, so during these workouts I would often push my body the extra mile. I had a Rocky Balboa like mindset; I felt I represented the words "Never give up" perfectly.

Besides feeling amazing, I was in an incredible mood. All the working out I was putting in was starting to affect my mood as well. My endorphins were in super concentrated mode and were being heavily utilized to the nth degree. People that knew me were never certain since I was usually the strong silent type. I rarely displayed emotion, but trust me I was unbelievably elated at this time. Despite some obstacles that happened during my junior year of high school all my hard work seemed to be paying off. My future was looking extremely bright.

This week was senior week where most high school seniors where I was from would take a trip down to Ocean City, Maryland for a week. They went down to celebrate the finale of their high school days. I was a junior going into my senior year, and this meant at work I would be getting more hours. Not as exciting as partying with my best friends at the beach but on the positive side it meant more money. Besides sports, I have always been motivated by success. While most kids growing up would think of random things while taking a shower, I was always constantly thinking of how I could make money. I was usually envisioning how I could be successful when I grew up.

Not only this, but at the pool I worked at there was three different pools. There was a baby pool, the lap pool, and the big main pool. I started lifeguarding when I was 15, so this was my third year at the Antietam Valley Recreation Community Center or "AVRCC", as we would call it. I had worked my way past the baby pool to the lap pool but was not very often scheduled to be on the big main pool. Being that this week was senior week that would change. The big main pool would be mine to guard. Here was my chance to shine in front of my managers and coworkers. If you knew me well, one thing you knew was I took pride in everything I did. I strived to make those I loved and respected proud.

This was sometimes to a fault as sometimes I could be overly self-conscious and come off shy in order make good impressions. If I had one fear it would be I sometimes may not have been outgoing enough, or afraid I might rub someone the wrong way if I was.

The day started out wonderful. Weather was nice and work was going smooth. Between 2-3pm I decided to swim some laps and do some push-ups. With working at a pool, I decided that swimming would be my new cardio. I enjoyed swimming. It was something I did competitively for many years until I was 15 when I quit to play basketball full time. This was not an easy decision, one many people often questioned. The summer before I quit I had just placed 3rd in the county for 100m breast stroke for my age group. Some thought if I kept up with swimming I would be on pace to earn a scholarship.

After another successful swimming workout for cardio at the pool I felt hyped. After every successful workout, I kept getting more enthusiastic and thinking positively about the future. I was imagining what all my coaches and teammates would think when they saw how much my athletic abilities had improved. I often fantasized what my female classmates might think about my hard body. I was never a ladies man so the thought of getting some attention was exciting. I was never fat but I was born very skinny with a fast metabolism. I had a six pack at the time but one thing I always wanted to do was add some more muscle, which I was slowly starting to develop.

A couple hours later, out of nowhere I began to feel very fatigued. I was not sure why. I did not think it was that big of a deal. I figured since I had been working out so hard that my body just needed some time for rest and recovery. So, I reacted how any normal person would. During my break, down from the lifeguard chair, I put a cold towel over my head, closed my eyes and got a quick nap in before my next shift up. I figured the rest would help me feel a little bit better.

I indeed dozed off for a little bit. I was glad to get a quick nap. The rest was much needed. Once I woke up it was just about time for my shift up on the lifeguard chair. In fact, I had just about a minute to spare. I had napped longer than I anticipated. My walk to the lifeguard chair to switch shifts did not feel any different than any time before. At first I did not realize anything was wrong. It was not until up on the chair I realized something very strange was happening. As a lifeguard, a given habit we did was swing and twirls our whistles around in our hand while on the chair. As I started winding my whistle around my hand, I realized something was very abnormal. It was such a strange sensation. Immediately, I recognized something did not feel right at all. I could not figure out what it was at first. I then began to realize though, that when I would twirl my whistle it was like I could not feel my arms in space. It was like I lost a sense of gravity. I have never been up in space but I imagined this is what it might feel like. I became very lightheaded and my heart slightly began to race. I had no clue what in the world was going on. I was scared and began to slightly panic. I kept thinking to myself *what I should do*? At first I thought about double whistling to make it seem if someone was drowning to draw attention. To let my coworkers know I needed help and to possibly call an ambulance. My first reaction was that I could be having a heart attack.

No matter how scared I was, my pride at the time would not let me call for help. Instead I kept acting like nothing was wrong. I did not want to disappoint my managers nor embarrass myself in front of my coworkers. I had always tried to come off and portray myself as the quiet tough guy and I was not about to stop now. I kept

13

thinking and began telling myself it was just anxiety. Hoping this would make the bizarre symptoms disappear. Anxiety attacks were something I had before. It was a possibility it could be happening again. I was not sure why. I was not nervous about anything. My attitude was positive. I was in great spirits. However, I was underneath a lot of stress. Since I was in a good mood I felt the stress was not affecting me. There was always the possibility of being wrong.

My mom had just recently broken her leg. With her recovering from a broken leg and me being the oldest sibling, it meant more responsibilities and things I had to take care of around the house. I had to help take care of my brother and sister. A lot of the things that my mother did that I took for granted now became some of my responsibility. Still to the best of my knowledge I had felt like I was handling everything very well.

Halfway through my half hour shift, dark clouds started to roll in and a loud bang of thunder occurred. My coworker whistled for thunder and told everyone to clear the pool. I could not have been more relieved. With the way I was feeling I could not wait to get down off the chair. To make it even better, the forecast showed the weather was not going to let up. It was already after 6pm and with the pool closing in a little over an hour, my managers decided to make the decision to close down the pool for the rest of the day. It would be an early dismissal.

I got my driver's license as early I could in Pennsylvania. I got my permit the day after my 16th birthday and took my driver's test the second I was able to. Being a new driver I enjoyed driving and having the freedom like most seventeen-year-olds. Except, this day driving home from work was different. I had never been more scared in my short diving career. I thought about calling my house to see if my step dad would have been able to pick me up but with my mom needing attention with her broken leg I did not want to cause more stress on the family. As soon as I pulled out the parking lot I could not wait until I got home. I still was not feeling right. Thankfully I somehow made it home okay. The pool I worked at was only 5 minutes away from my house but on this day the drive felt like a solid 20 minutes ride despite the fact I drove incredibly fast and not focused at all. I was an incredible liability on the roads. Needless to say, I made it home safe and that's all that mattered.

As I arrived at my house I kept wondering what I was going to tell my mom and step dad about how I was feeling. Things were already stressful and I did not want to add any more to the plate. I decided to be honest and let them know I was not feeling right but just blew it off like it was no big deal. I insisted I just needed to sleep it off. That night I did everything I normally did. I ate leftovers and helped my mom with her physical therapy exercises. The only difference was instead of being a night owl I went to bed right away.

Since nothing serious happened since everything strange started happening to my body earlier, I was having a slightly different outlook. By the time I was going to bed I was starting to become more convinced that I was probably just having a long anxiety attack. I assumed I would just go to sleep and wake up feeling back to normal.

Like most people, I woke up between 3-4am in the middle of the night; unfortunately, this was going to be different than any other night. The one thing not the same was I had to pee really bad. Laugh if you want but believe it or not this was unusual for me. My mother and brother grew up with weak bladders and were known to have to urinate regularly through the night but not me. I was known to have a strong bladder. My mom used to refer to me as having a "Bladder of steel". My bladder of steel was not going let this urge go, so even though I dreaded getting up, I got out of bed and headed to the bathroom.

Little did I know this would turn out to be the "Piss from Hell". As I started pissing, my heart started flying and I mean it was flying. I played sports my whole life. I ran 3.1 miles for cross country but my heart was racing faster than it would after a cross country race. At seventeen-years-old I truly believed I was having a heart attack, this time there was almost no doubt in my mind. Why in the world would my heart be pounding and racing like this just for standing up to go pee. I was petrified again but still determined to not make it a big deal or cause a scene. I kept thinking to myself that there was no way I could be having a heart attack no matter how real it felt. There is no way something serious could be happening to me. I was too young and healthy. With my mom breaking her leg I do not have time for anything serious, nor does my family. I kept trying to brush it off like everything was going to be okay. I was convinced this had to be just a bad dream. I could not possibly be awake right now; this has to be a nightmare. I wanted to believe once I made it back to my bed, fell back asleep; I would wake up with everything back to ordinary.

There was one big problem; I never made it back to my bed. As I took a couple steps out of the bathroom, everything went black. I was blacking out for the first time in my life. It was like seeing my life flash before my eyes. So finally, out of life and death fear I collapsed to the ground with my hands over my head. With the little breath and energy, I had remaining, I screamed for help.

Miraculously, Once I hit the floor and after I screamed, light started coming back. I began to see again. Not very well, as things were still blurry, but at least everything was not completely black. Fortunately, my step dad heard me screaming. I could hear him making his way up the steps. Once he came up he asked what happened. I explained everything. I informed him of my racing heart, to almost blacking out, feeling light headed and tremendously weak. He helped me get back to my bed and told me to try and get a good night sleep. He told me that later in the morning we would visit the doctor.

I agreed but after everything that had just transpired I could not fall back asleep. I just lied down in my bed trying to stay positive. Thinking of ways and techniques to relax myself and calm down my nerves. The problem is I was terrified. I had no clue what was going on with my body but at this point I could almost guarantee it was not anxiety related. To make it worse I kept having flashbacks. Earlier in the year on March 15th one of my best friends Joshua Wayne Anthony Brown passed away. He collapsed playing basketball and the cause of his death was determined to be from an enlarged heart. Two years earlier a basketball teammate Jordan Jermacans, a grade below me passed away on the team bus during a trip to a game. He had a violent seizure. Just like my friend Josh, his death was determined to be caused by an enlarged heart. Unlike most people my age, I had witnessed that even the youngest, fittest, athletic and seemingly the healthiest can die young to heart related illnesses. I was just praying I was not the next one. Family history was not in my favor. My mother had a heart murmur and my grandmother had heart disease. The one thing that kept me positive was that I was still alive and lying down my heart rate was back to normal. Knowing I was going to the doctor the next day encouraged me as well. I was assured they would find out what was wrong. I was under the impression I would be on the road to recovery soon.

The Mystery

As I was getting ready to go see the doctor I knew something with my body still was not right. Nothing had changed from the moment I stepped up on that lifeguard chair the day before. Whenever I went to the doctor in the past, the wait never seemed that bad. If I went to the doctor it was usually just for an annual physical. The physical usually ended up with the doctors raving about how healthy I was. If I did go to the doctor for other things such as cold, at least I knew it was nothing tremendously serious. I was just going to get prescribed antibiotics to take care of my illness. Knowing that once it would kick in within a week I would be back to my old self

This time was different. The wait to see the doctor seemed like forever. What I was experiencing literally made me feel like I was about to die. It was like I was going to wither away. That I was going to gradually become so weak I couldn't move my limbs. I stayed lightheaded and dizzy no matter what I did. My heart kept racing when I was not lying down and I was exhausted. I could not concentrate, had no appetite and the weirdest feeling of all was the feeling as if I was floating. Like I lost sense of gravity, my arms were like feathers. I felt so light that a strong push of wind could make me float me away.

Once the doctor called me in I figured I would get some type of news whether good or bad. I assumed they would at least order some type of tests that should be done to try and explain what was going on. I slowly began to explain to the doctor what had just happened to me to the best of my ability. This was difficult since I was extremely tired and did not feel like I had complete control of my breathing. As I started to explain what I was feeling, to my surprise the doctor seemed completely unconcerned. She took my pulse sitting down. It was normal just like everything else except for my blood pressure being a little high. She proceeded to tell me that it is normal to get a racing heart when getting up to go the bathroom in the middle of the night. She even gave a technical term that is used to describe this, though I cannot remember it to this day nor find anything on google when I researched. As for the blood pressure, chest pain and the loss of feeling, she contributed these issues to be caused by anxiety. The general weakness she determined was most likely a viral infection. She ordered me to follow up with a neurologist and cardiologist but she was convinced nothing was wrong.

I do not recall ever feeling as hopeless as I did coming back from the doctor that day. Deep in my gut I knew something was not right but I was being told otherwise. The only instructions I was given was to rest and drink lots of fluids.

For the next week rest is what I sure did. I rarely got off the couch. The only time I felt normal was when I was lying down. As soon as I started to stand up is when all hell would begin to break loose. Upon standing, all the symptoms that I have described before would start to act up. During this week I also followed up with the cardiologist and neurologist. They did as many tests as you can imagine from blood tests, MRI, x-rays, to wearing a heart monitor. With all these tests being done I finally felt like something was going to be discovered. I was certain they had to find something that was causing me to feel this way. Again I was wrong. All the tests came back perfect. In fact, the cardiologist went as far as saying "That I was healthy as a horse, all the tests looked unremarkable and at seventeen I was too young to have any heart problems." To most seventeen-year-olds this would be reassuring but for me it was not. Just witnessing one of my closest friends at seventeen die of enlarged heart made me very aware that even though the chances are rare, that heart issues can happen even in the young and fit.

Once the results came back, my family figured I had to be fine. They insisted that after a week of lying around it was time to get up start living my life and push through it. They thought this would be best for me and help get over my viral infection. At the time, all I had been diagnosed with was a viral infection so this is what everyone suspected I had. So, I tried to get out. I was scared because I did not feel right but all the tests were saying nothing was wrong with me. I did not believe that anxiety could cause me to feel the way I did but I thought who knows maybe the doctor and my family were right. Maybe if I go about my normal life then my body will go back to feeling normal.

I tried going back to work. I started lifeguarding again but I was not always able to make it through the days. There were a couple times I had called my friends to pick me up and take me home. As time was going by things were getting more difficult. My work had no idea what was up with me and all my friends and family had no idea what was going on with me either. Everyone just seemed to believe I was just suffering from severe anxiety.

All of this was getting to me. Whenever people asked what was wrong all I could do was tell them I'm not sure, I don't feel well or it is something with my heart. Some people were scared for me others thought I was losing it or again thought I was just suffering from severe anxiety. Besides not feeling well I was suffering from depression. I once took pride in being the strong silent type but now I felt weak, both mentally and physically. I have always been quiet but I was always still very confident. Not anymore. At this moment in my life I felt extremely insecure. It felt as if I was being judged and constantly talked behind my back. I saw friends and coworkers that used to hang around me a lot start to distance themselves from me. I no longer felt as respected as I once thought I might have been. Instead, I sensed I was becoming an outcast. I even started to question if I was totally with it. Thoughts would occasionally cross my mind if it was worth still living if this was how my life was going to be from now on. Every day was becoming a struggle both physically and mentally. Life was not fun anymore. I was given no answers. There seemed to be very little light at the end of the tunnel.

Despite having suicidal thoughts, I am proud to say I never acted upon them. Even though I often felt hopeless, I always had this tiny hope inside me that I would eventually cross paths with a doctor who would find out what was wrong. I kept dreaming that one day I would live a normal life again. I would often dream that I would feel healthy and get back to being the same old person I used to be. I often looked back at the past, wishing I could go back.

I contribute this tiny bit of hope to how I have been wired ever since I was young. Ever since I was a young kid I always believed I was going to be somebody one day and I would accomplish great things. I truly believed that, I felt like I was meant to be someone. As if I was destined to do something great. Maybe I'm right or maybe I'm wrong, whatever it is, that belief is what has kept me alive. This belief is what has made me achieve everything I have accomplished up to this point in my life. This belief is what gave me the slightest bit of hope when I felt hope was all gone.

My mental and physical situation was taking a toll inside my household. I ended up in the emergency room in the beginning of July and again they found nothing wrong. I still kept complaining that I did not feel right and for the last time my step dad decided to take me to the doctor's office again. This was worse than any other time. It was a waste of visit. No tests were ordered. In fact, nothing was done at all. Basically, I went in, he checked my pulse sitting down, and then he checked my blood pressure, just like a normal routine checkup. After two minutes, he told me I was fine. He was very stern and came off as he was one hundred percent sure I was having anxiety. He was rude and did not seem to care for me very much. He told me I needed to get myself together. He made it very clear he thought I was not with it mentally. What he did do was prescribe me anxiety medication for a couple days.

After this appointment, I did not know what else to do. I was embarrassed. I took the anxiety medication and it did not change how I felt at all. Yes, it calmed my nerves but it did not take the racing heart away or my loss of sensation. My limbs still felt like feathers. The doctor's advice and diagnosis reassured people that everything I was going through was anxiety. It was tough. When I would go places and people found out that I was having anxiety issues, they would tell me such things like 'It is okay, we all have stress." They would let me know "Not to worry, it will get better." Some would joke how I was too young to have stress at seventeen and that the stress will only get worse as I get older. I ignored these comments and tried to brush them off, but deep down, these comments hurt. It felt like I was being portrayed as an outcast of society. I started to even question if I was, but deep down I knew I was not an outcast. I knew what I was feeling was real. I began to wish I could trade places with people so they could experience what I was going through. I never wanted to wish horrible things on anyone, but I just wanted people to understand what I was going through. I wanted them to know how it felt to feel like every day you were fighting for your life. Only to be told you are crazy. Everyday, I was fighting to keep my heart rate down, to get rid of chest pain, fighting to not get weaker, and fighting to regain sensation and feeling in my limbs again. I so desperately just wanted people to understand and see how limited my quality of life was despite how healthy I might have looked on the outside. They say P.O.T.S. is an invisible disease and I sure could have not felt anymore invisible to people.

The stress my situation was putting on my household finally hit its boiling point between early to mid August. It got to the point that I was told to leave. I was told to leave not because they did not love me, they made it very clear they still did very much but because they thought it was best for everyone in the family. It was too much for everyone to handle with both my mom and my quality of life being extremely limited at the time. Plus, they were tired of me being not pushing through what they believed at the time was just anxiety. They were tired of me not taking their advice on how to get better. They felt like I was jeopardizing my job and my future. It was becoming too much and they could no longer take time out to spend money and keep taking me on doctors' visits just to keep hearing the same thing by a different doctor reiterating I was hundred percent normal. At this point I had not been diagnosed with anything. Numerous doctors just told me I was having anxiety and to get over it.

With my mom's broken leg, times in our household were already hard enough without adding my issues. My step-dad had to try and work from home. He sacrificed and did this while still trying to make enough money to pay the bills, put food on the table and take care of my mother. Being the older sibling I was supposed to step up and help with home chores but with my health, I was making things more difficult. Now my fourteen-year-old brother would have to step up which is asking a lot of fourteen-year-old, plus he cannot drive which was I was supposed to help out with so I could make sure that he and my sister would get to where they needed to go. Now that was another burden put on my step-dad's shoulders.

I was upset, angry, hopeless, and felt terrible. When I first heard my mom broke her leg, it was a voicemail from my step-dad. I heard it on my way home from school. I remember after I heard the voicemail I just screamed in my car while I was stopped at a stoplight. I could not understand why this had to happen to my mom. My mom was such an important part of our family. She did and sacrificed so much for us and I knew her being out of commission was going to take such a toll on the family. I was devastated but I knew I could not change things so I decided I would embrace it and make the most of it. I always claimed to be the strong silent type and in adversity I wanted to show I could handle more responsibilities. I wanted to make my mom proud. I always viewed myself as a leader and I wanted to show my brother and sister how to lead by example. Before that day on June 16th I was doing just that. I was doing so much that my mom would often tell me that maybe I should rest a little bit. She thought I often looked tired. She would constantly tell me I had dark circles underneath my eyes. I refused to. That was not in my DNA. I was not a quitter. I was motivated and I wanted to show my family and everyone else I can handle and accomplish anything when facing adversity.

Two months later and now I am packing up my bags. I was speechless. I never pictured the day I would be told to leave. I understood where they were coming from but I was still upset not just with them but also myself. I could not understand why my body felt the way it did. I so desperately wanted to feel normal again. I was tired of living every day scared like it was going to be my last but I could not prevent it. No matter what I did or how much anxiety medication I took, this is how my body felt.

I called my dad and told him what was going on. My mom and dad divorced before I was even a year old so I never knew what it was like when they were together. Divorced life was all I knew. I spent majority of the time with my mom growing up and would see my dad whenever he had off from work. He was a police officer for the city of Reading. Throughout my life, I was used to him picking me up to visit but this time was different. Once he picked me up I had no idea when I would see my mom, brother, sister, or step-dad again. I had no idea what was going to happen. We all cried when I walked out when my dad picked me up. In fact, I cried almost that whole night. I felt more hopeless than I had ever been; even more than the times I would come back from the doctors and they would tell me nothing was wrong. No one believed in me. No one believed that I was actually sick. They all thought it was in my head. For the first time in my life I felt completely alone. I was empty. I thought of just giving up on life, and put some serious thought into it. At this point I figured not many people would care. All I was, was someone that created more stress and problems. Everyone was getting frustrated with me and no one believed how I was actually feeling. It was as if I had no worth and was worthless. Life to me did not seem to have a purpose. The past couple months I have just been a pain in the ass.

After all the negative thoughts ran through my head, I started to realize something. To this day, I am not sure what came over me but I started to have a change of heart. I realized there was *someone* that believed in me. I knew my body better than anyone else and I believed in myself. I thought to myself, I do not need anyone to believe in me. I believe in me. Again, I do not know what came across me but that night after all the tears went away I decided I am going to do whatever it takes to figure out what's going on, even if it means I have to do it all on my own. One way or another I was going to get my life back. Deep down I still had this tiny bit of hope that believed I was meant to do something in life. There was no way this was how my life was going to end. Not me, I was meant to be somebody someday.

The Diagnosis

Staying with my dad did not mean he had a different perception of me than anyone else. He was also positive I was just suffering from anxiety. The only difference was he did not have a broken leg or anyone else to take care of. To him I was the only child, so even though he did not believe anything was seriously wrong, he would still help me if need be, or at least I thought.

Two days went by and I did not hear anything from anyone. Despite lying on the couch all day resting and watching TV I was not getting better. In fact, I kept getting worse. Whenever I stood up, the dizzier I got, the faster my heart would race. I felt like I was about to faint.

Growing up my dad was not the easiest person to talk to. He was the strong silent type just like me. At times he could come off like he did not want to be bothered. In spite of being a little nervous to approach him about how terrified I was about my current health situation; I did anyway. I asked for him to take me to the doctor again. At first, he was not so sure. He told me that I have already been to the doctor several times and was not sure what else they could do for me. I knew where he was coming from but I knew my body better than anyone else. Regardless from what the doctors have been saying, I knew they were wrong. I was positive something was not right with my body. For me to act like this was not like me at all. Finally, after my father began to see how persistent I was on that something was wrong and he could tell how poor my quality of life was becoming, he caved in. He called up the doctor's office and made an appointment for the next day.

As I woke up the next morning, my dad and I headed out to the doctor's office. I was not quite sure how to feel. I could tell he was irritated we were even doing this but deep down inside I knew this trip had to be made. I just kept hoping I would get a different doctor. A doctor that for once we would get me some answers, answers I have been seeking for almost three months now.

After a half hour of waiting in the doctor's office, the doctor finally arrived. His name was Dr. Raymond Hubbard. He was a middle-aged doctor and had a very intelligent almost professor like look to him. He was in shape, had glasses and had a thick but trimmed goatee. Besides working at the local Reading Pediatrics office in Reading, PA he was widely respected and would help out in Africa with patients. Actually, he just recently won the "Russell S. Bickel Jr. Award for Excellence in Communication and Caring to Patients and Their Families."

This was the first time I had met Dr. Hubbard. I had no idea how well respected he was until I started to get to know him better. Even still, being the first time meeting him, there was something about his whole demeanor that made me believe I was starting to feel like I might finally get an answer. As I explained to Dr. Hubbard how I had been feeling the past couple months and everything that had happened, it was almost like I could see his brain moving and analyzing everything. He did the normal routine checkup and started to ask some more follow up questions. After all questions were asked there was nothing but silence. You could tell he was thinking very hard. His wheels were turning. Finally, he looked up at me and told me he wanted to check my heart rate and blood pressure in three different positions. One was lying down, the other sitting up and the last one was standing up. This is known as the tilt table test. These were orthostatic blood pressure measurements. A tilt table test does orthostatic plus cardio and oxygen monitoring while lying on a table that can be shifted and adjusted into different angles. Believe it or not out of all the times I had previously visited the doctors or ended up in the emergency room at the Reading Hospital this was a test that had never been performed yet.

After the tilt table test was completed. Dr. Hubbard glanced at my results. His eyes began to light up. He then proceeded to tell me he believed he knew what the problem was. He said "I'm afraid you have what is called P.O.T.S. I replied "POTS?" I had never heard of it and the name was very strange. It made me think of pots and pans or flower pots. He said "Yes- P.O.T.S.". He went on to explain how it was an acronym for Postural Orthostatic Tachycardia Syndrome. He let me know that my heart rate when lying down was perfectly normal around 60 beats per minute. But when I was standing my heart would raise up to 130 beats per minute without walking which was way higher than what a normal person's should be. This would explain all the racing heart and chest pain symptoms. It also explained for my fatigue and shortness of breath. Dr. Hubbard also went on to explain how this is a dysautonomia disease and my body is not reacting well to gravity which also explained my loss of sensation and floating feeling.

At first when I heard this I was actually terrified. I had never heard of this syndrome. I had so many thoughts racing through my head. Am I going to eventually die? Is this curable? How long will I have it? Am I at great risk for a heart attack? What even caused me to get this crazy dysautonomia disorder?

Dr. Hubbard went on to explain how P.O.T.S. is a new phenomenon and is being researched more and more as an increasingly amount of more people are being diagnosed. He explained there are many causes but a particular cause was not known. Some of the causes are stress, concussions, pregnancy, puberty, or a viral infection which is what may have caused mine. He informed me that some may recover (which has been highly questioned) while others it will remain with them their whole life. He stated that this syndrome can be severely crippling and have a huge impact on your quality of life at times. He also made it very clear that P.O.T.S. has not been linked to cause any deaths or heart problems as of the time being. He did mention that a lot of research is still being done. He instructed me to drink lots of fluids and to rest and that he would see me again soon to discuss a plan to help relieve and manage my symptoms. He was very optimistic that he could get me back on the road to recovery.

Once I got home, my dad started researching more about P.O.T.S. (Postural Orthostatic Tachycardia Syndrome). This was something that neither of us had ever heard of before. The more he learned and shared with me, the more certain we knew that Dr. Hubbard was right in his diagnosis. All my symptoms and issues matched up perfectly with the descriptions of P.O.T.S. we found online.

P.O.T.S is known by very few in the United States but believe it or not today between one to three million Americans are currently affected with this syndrome. In order to be diagnosed with P.O.T.S. your body must show an increase of heart rate of at least 30 beats per minute when standing up or a heart rate of 120 beats per minute or higher. These readings must be done within ten minutes of standing and determined by a tilt table test. Most P.O.T.S. patients have a significant drop in blood pressure while standing though some have even shown to increase.

P.O.T.S. was discovered by a collective group of researchers at the Mayo Clinic which was led by Neurologist Dr. Phillip Low. Before 1993, all symptoms of P.O.T.S. were believed by doctors to be just anxiety but after much extensive research they discovered this was not the case. Research has proven that P.O.T.S. is not caused by anxiety but is actually caused by a malfunction of the patient's autonomic nervous system making it a dysutonomia disorder. We looked to see if there was any specialist in this syndrome but the closest one at the time was Dr. Blair Grub at the University of Toledo Medical Center. We made a call to Dr. Grubb but there was a waiting list to see him that was almost a year long. This was back in 2008. As of today, the waiting list to see Dr. Blair Grubb is two years long.

P.O.T.S. is unique in the sense it causes such an array of symptoms. There is still no complete cure. Each person affected by P.O.T.S. may show a vast array of different complicated symptoms. Besides an increase in heart rate, P.O.T.S. can cause nausea, extreme fatigue, headache, shortness of breath, fainting, light headiness, heart palpitations, coldness or pain in extremities, poor circulation, loss of sensation, chest pain, neuropathy and many more. Upon research, many studies have shown that these symptoms caused 25 percent of people not to be able to work. Only 18.2 percent of P.O.T.S. patients have fully recovered and 52.8 percent improved symptoms and their quality of life but have never completely recovered. According to the research there are multiple medications that can try and treat P.O.T.S. patients but the main thing was just living a healthy lifestyle. Medications can help but will only help relieve or manage symptoms if you continue to eat a healthy diet and get some form of exercise. Again, this is all based on a variety of research. As you will learn later every person and doctor seems to have a different belief on certain aspects of P.O.T.S.

After first being diagnosed with P.O.T.S. and going over all the information my dad had found out about this bizarre syndrome, I was not quite sure how to feel. I was relieved to know that my condition was not life threatening but I was extremely disappointed in the fact I was not sure how long I would be dealing with this syndrome nor how quickly my symptoms would improve. How I felt and the thought of conquering this syndrome was overwhelming. The realization began setting in that things were going to be different. I began to think how I was going to be able to make it through my senior year of high school and would I be able to play high school sports again? What were my fellow classmates and teachers going to think of me? How would my respective coaches respond to the news? How was I going to explain what was wrong with me? I now had a diagnosis but one that was so unheard of and hard to understand. Were people still going to look at me like I'm crazy?

I could tell my dad was having a hard time with the diagnosis as well. No one wants to see their kid suffer but he kept encouraging me everything was going to be alright. As the next couple days went by I was good in the sense that I no longer was having the fear that I may be dying but I obviously still felt horrible. I rested a lot and drank a tremendous amount of fluids. Whenever I felt up to it I would do research on my new profound illness and watched any video I could of someone who was going through the same thing as I was. I finally gathered up the courage and called my cross-country coach to notify him of everything that what was going on with my health. Coach "Worm" as we used to call him was a great guy. I had much respect for him. He cared about each of his players personally but also had a fiery and competitive side to him for he desperately wanted to win. I was not sure how he was going to take the news being that close to the end of my junior year I was making constant improvement and figured to possibly be a key contributor to the team during my upcoming senior season. Luckily, Coach Worm was very understanding. He let me know I still had a roster spot on the team and that he would be willing to work with me on my medical issue. I next went and called the AVRCC where I was a lifeguard. This I was even more nervous about but I did have a doctor's note. Again, my manager was very understanding and reassured me that once the doctor cleared me to work I would have my job back. It made it easier that the AVRCC always had an abundance of lifeguards working for them. I was glad Coach Worm and my manager at the pool I lifeguarded at was very understanding. I do not think they completely understood what my diagnosis was or what I was going through but at most they thought it might have something to do with the heart, just like most other people.

Towards the end of the week my mom reached out to me. We talked. I apologized for getting upset and they apologized for everything that happened and were deeply saddened by my diagnosis. Just like my dad they could not believe this is something any of their children would have to go through. I moved back in with my mom and things were getting better as a family. My dad was still going to have to help me out a lot due to my mom's broken leg but he understood that. For once it felt good to have everyone's support during this difficult time. I still was overwhelmed at the fact how long it was going to take me to recover but for the first time in months I actually felt I was going to beat what was ever happening to my body. My spirits were lifted and my killer instincts kicked in. I was determined I was not going to lose this battle to P.O.T.S.

The Recovery

Now that my illness was finally determined, it was time to start putting action plans in place. I needed an organized plan in order to try and recover or put the P.O.T.S. in remission. The many people I needed to get in contact with were Dr. Hubbard, my cross-country coach, the nurse and counseling staff at my high school. It was now time to make the people aware what is going on in my life that are going to be needed in order for me to accomplish getting through my senior year of high school.

Before meeting with anyone else it was imperative that I first listened to what Dr. Hubbard had to say in my follow up appointment. In the follow up appointment we discussed my most problematic symptoms. He stressed the importance of getting the proper amount of sleep but to be careful of over sleeping. I was to get rest when needed but not over rest, He referred me for physical therapy. It would be both on land and in water. Aqua therapy would help my body with re adjusting to gravity. He encouraged me to keep up with drinking plenty of fluids and also prescribed a special salt tablet. Last but not least he wanted me to see someone who somewhat specialized in this new P.O.T.S. syndrome. The biggest and most known specialist was Dr. Grubb in Toledo, Ohio but that was a little far for me and the waiting list was long. So, he referred me to a doctor at Penn State Hershey Medical Center named Rachel Levine. She had some background with P.O.T.S. Dr. Hubbard thought it was best to be seen by two doctors to get more than one view to see if they had other advice. Everything at this visit was sounding positive until he brought up about me possibly being able to participate in high school sports for my senior year. He was realistic with me and stated that cross-country and basketball were most definitely out of the question but depending on my recovery I could possibly recover enough to be cleared to play volleyball. He could not guarantee anything. It would be a quicker recovery than most but we were determined to make that the goal and beat the odds. He told me how some people take years to get better and others within 6 months. But most research at this time stated it would take years. Usually symptoms decrease as you entered into mid adulthood. We both agreed that to be cleared to participate in volleyball during the spring would be our main goal. Volleyball was my favorite sport in High School. Our team won State in 2007, and the past season I went on a visit to St. Francis, PA University to meet with the coach to discuss the opportunity of possibly playing volleyball there. At the time, I was told that he did not have a scholarship available for me but the idea of joining the team as a practice player and working my way up was a possibility. For those unaware, there are only four colleges in Pennsylvania that carry men's volleyball as an NCAA sport and just not a club sport. So to even be offered that opportunity was exciting.

After hearing this news, I was saddened that I would miss out on two sports but it was something I was expecting. It did however motivate me more than ever. I wanted to beat this and be able to participate in volleyball for my senior season. To me that would be a win. I wanted to be the rare exception and improve within months from my syndrome. There was no way I was going to let this thing go on for years.

After the follow up with Dr. Hubbard the next step was to contact Coach Worm my cross-country coach and let him know the disappointing news. After telling Coach Worm the news I could tell he was disappointed and felt bad for me. He did agree to still let me be part of the team and support them. He also advised me to get in contact with our school's athletic trainer to set up a special training

35

program for me after school that I could participate in while the team practiced after school. Telling Coach Worm I would not be able to run with the team this year was extremely difficult but I was relieved that he was so willing to help me out with everything that was going on. I did what he told me and I contacted Audrey our high school's athletic trainer and notified her of my condition. "P.O.T.S." This syndrome unfortunately was something new to her. She informed me she would do as much research as possible on the condition and reassured me once school started she would have my own after school workout plan to help me.

Now was the hard part. My mom got in contact with the school and explained to them my situation. After my mom told them everything that was going on, we scheduled a meeting with the school guidance counselor and nurse to figure out a program to cater to my needs once the school year started. During this meeting the counselor made me aware that I had the right to go to the school nurse whenever I wanted and she would notify all my teachers of this. The school also allowed me to have a key to the elevator whenever I felt like walking up the steps would be too much. The nurse told me she would meet with me every day and I was allowed in her office whenever I was not feeling well. Every day we were to meet so she could record readings of my blood pressure and heart rate both sitting and standing. These would then be sent over to my family doctor every time I followed up with him so he could see how I was progressing.

Meeting and informing the school was definitely embarrassing. Relying on other people and having these special privileges made me feel weak; however I knew it had to be done. I was more nervous for the school year to start as it was only two weeks away. I had no idea how I would make it through the school day and was uncomfortable as to what my peers would think when they saw I was completely out of it. I knew I would be questioned whenever I had to use the elevator because I could not make it up the steps. Whenever I had a P.O.T.S. attack, when symptoms would get severe it could come off as I was on some hard drugs. I could just imagine all the rumors that could start spreading about me because of my new diagnosed illness.

Despite how nervous I was, one thing that had to be done was to see the doctor up at Penn State Hershey. I had never been to Penn State Hershey but I heard many great things about it. It ranked as one of the best hospitals in the country. The doctor I ended up seeing Rachel Levine eventually would get promoted and now works as the physician general for the Commonwealth of Pennsylvania. However, the first day I met her I was confused. Her main focus was working primarily with children with eating disorders. This did not mean she knew nothing about P.O.T.S. Again, she is regarded as one of the most knowledgeable doctors in the state but it still threw me off guard. At this point I was still hoping there was some magical news that there may be a quick recovery, so I went in with an open mind. The meeting did not go as I hoped. She knew a lot about P.O.T.S. but did not really inform me of anything new that Dr. Hubbard had not already told me. The one thing this doctor did was prescribe me depression medication. She thought it would be a good idea since she could tell the news of having P.O.T.S. was dragging me down.

I started following all my doctor's orders. It had only been a little over a week but I had not noticed any difference yet in how I was feeling. Not only that but today was my first day of my senior year of high school and the first day I was going to school with severe P.O.T.S. It started off unusual as I was dropped off at my bus stop by my step dad. Being a senior and having my license I usually drove to school and if I did have to take the bus I usually walked but now the walk would have been too much for me to handle. The bus stop was a bit of a walk and one that would make me go up a little hill in the neighborhood. It was embarrassing but again something I had to do. With my physical health at the time I had no other options. Once I got to school I had tremendous anxiety. My high school had a little over 1,000 people in it and being around all these people was intimidating especially the way I was feeling. I had this picture that everyone would be staring at me but this was not case. One of the hardest things about P.O.T.S. is even though I'm extremely sick on the inside; you still look perfectly fine on the outside. A lot of times I felt like people could tell when I was not feeling well but that was not always necessarily true. I never knew invisible diseases existed until I was diagnosed with one. And to be honest it sucked. At times, you are literally invisible to everyone. You could feel like you are on the verge of fainting and no one would even notice.

I made it through first period fine but just as second period started I was already tired and could not wait to lie down. I knew this was going to be hard but this was the first time I realized how hard it was going to be to make it through the school day. At home, whenever I started not to feel well I could lie down on a couch right away but it would not be that easy in school. Despite how tired I was I was determined I was not going to ask to go to the nurse's office at the beginning of second period. I was not ready to be embarrassed yet.

By the time third period rolled around for a double period of British Literature I was regretting not going to the nurse's office to rest. I was completely exhausted. I was still so determined not to go to the nurse's office but I had to do something. My body could no longer even sit up straight, I was feeling horrible. So, I ended up putting my head down on my desk and started to rest. It looked just like I was sleeping. I did not know how the teacher would respond but he had to be aware of my illness because he did not say anything and I know if I had done something like that in the past he would have approached me about it. After the period was over one of my close friends came up to me and started laughing. He could not believe I was almost sleeping in class on the first day. He was not laughing in a bad way however he almost thought it was cool. He thought I was trying to be a rebel. I did not tell him the real reason why I was almost sleeping. I was not ready yet for him to know, so instead, I just smiled in acknowledgement.

Next was lunch. At lunch, I sat down with my friends. I did not say much at all. In fact, I laid my head down and started sleeping on the lunch table. My friends started laughing and were wondering what was up. They were busting my balls and thought I was really high. Again, I was not ready to tell them what was wrong so I just played it off and told them I did not get much sleep the night before. The looks on their faces made it seem like if they were not sure whether to believe me or not but either way after a while they finally decided to let it go.

After lunch was 5th period. I walked into fifth period and I was not sure how I even made it there. As soon as I sat down my heart was flying. After five minutes into the class and once the teacher handed out the syllabus I approached her and asked her if I could head down to the nurses office. I was embarrassed and did not want to do it but my body could no longer take anymore. Fortunately, my teacher was Ms. Siedel at time who taught Contemporary Issues. She was very nice and understanding. She let me know she was notified of everything by the schools guidance team of what was going on with my health and told me to get on my way.

As soon as I got down to the nurse, she could tell I was out of it. You cannot always tell when a person with P.O.T.S. is not feeling up to par but the nurse could tell right away something was not right with me. She encouraged me to lie down ASAP. After lying down for a while the nurse finally approached me and asked how the day was going and how I was feeling. I explained everything that was going on. We recorded my orthostatic results and she advised me I could stay in her office and rest as long as I needed too. I felt horrible and I honestly just wanted to stay there and rest the rest of the school day but I did not want to miss any of my other classes. One exciting thing about the first day of class is getting to see who is going to be in your class. So, once it was time to go to 6th period I got the courage to stand up and walk to my next class. On the way out the nurse's office, Mrs. Duffner let me know to come back down if need be.

Once in 6th period I felt a little better now that I got to rest but I still could not wait for the day to be over. Unfortunately, this aura of feeling a little bit better did not last long at all. As 6th period was coming to a close I could barely keep my eyes open. I was determined I was not going to go back down to the nurse's office again. As determined as I was my body had other plans. Ten minutes into the beginning of 7th period my heart started flying again and this time I felt if I did not get rest soon I was going to faint or collapse. I was terrified so I listened to my body. I caved in and asked my teacher to go to the nurse again. My teacher Mrs. McGaffin who ended up being one of my all-time favorite teachers in high school, again, was very understanding and made it clear she also was notified of everything that was going on with my health.

As I entered the nurse's office for the second time that day, Mrs. Duffner was very friendly. I lied down right away and this time she encouraged me to stay until the end of the day. I had no problem abiding her advice. My last class for 8th period was a study hall, so I could care less if I missed that class. As I lied down in the nurses' office I started thinking of everything and started to tear up. Never in my whole life did I picture this would be how my first day of my senior year would start out. I was in shock. I sat there on the nurse's bed wanting so bad to get up and go back to class. I wanted to go after school and meet with my cross-country teammates and go for a run. This was the way it was supposed to be. Being my last year this was supposed to be special. I was having a hard time coming to grips with the fact my body would not allow this. I hated how ill I felt and I did not understand how or why this had to happen to me. As I mentioned previously, I was always the quiet type growing up and going through school. I was a guy of few words but I always had more than enough friends and was heavily involved with school activities. I was not the most popular person but I was no outcast either. One thing I never felt was alone but for the first time in all my school life going all the way back to kindergarten, I felt alone. Here I was the first day of my senior year spending the rest of the day lying down in the nurse's office all alone in a school full of over one thousand students feeling so distant from everything and everyone.

With the way I was feeling there was no way I could stay after school to learn about my special workout program with the athletic trainer Audrey Krause. I felt bad. Audrey was a nice lady. Knew her stuff and was extremely well liked by all the students. I just had no energy. So, I hopped aboard my school bus to head home. I had not ridden the school bus home since I had received my license and with the way I was feeling the ride home felt like an eternity. Not only that but with being the first day of school everyone was loud, excited and rowdy on the bus ride home which did not make me feel any better. The one thing I needed at this time was silence and rest.

Once the bus dropped me off, my step dad was right there to pick me up since I would not make it home walking over the little hills we had in our development. Once I got in the car he asked me how my day was and I explained how everything went. He could tell I look exhausted and needed rest. The school day had pushed my body further than it had any other day since I was diagnosed with P.O.T.S. I was so exhausted that later that night I did not even have the energy to stand up for a shower. I needed to use a shower stool to sit down. This ended up being a regular occurrence for me until my symptoms would improve.

As I lied in my bed trying to fall asleep that night, I am not really sure what came over me but in a day where I felt sad, disappointed, angry, and frustrated most of the day I began to think positive. Not sure why this always happened at night. I have always been a deep thinker and liked to free my mind at night, so this had to be the case. But the more I began to think the happier I began to feel that I made it through the day and I did not have to be sent home early or called to the hospital like I thought might happen. I did not know if I would improve upon my first day's performance, how long it would take to improve my symptoms, or if I would decline in my progress but one thing I did feel was satisfied. I was content with myself for making it through the school day.

The whole first week of school I had to see the nurse twice a day to rest and would never be able to stay after school to meet with the athletic trainer and see my cross-country teammates. This would slowly begin to change as the weeks went on. Over the next couple weeks, there were some days I would only have to see the nurse once a day. Some days I even had enough energy that I would meet with my athletic trainer and get to see my cross-country teammates after school as well. I began to go to the teams meets and film all our meets and events. I never was able to but my goal was to make an end of the season DVD video. I also started my aqua and land therapy twice a week. I was determined to push myself. I was exhausted by the end of the day but I kept hoping it was all part of the recovery process. I believed that if I kept getting the proper amount of rest during the day and sleep at night I would not have a setback.

I began to tell some of my closest friends what was going with me. I finally was feeling a little better and decided it was time. Some I just explained it had something to do with the heart, others I told them it was Postural Orthostatic Tachycardia Syndrome (P.O.T.S.). Either way they never really seemed to comprehend it but at the end of the day they supported me. I am sure there were times were I was being judged but after a while I stopped being embarrassed and caring what others thought. I no longer was doing things to impress my peers, I was in survival mode. I needed to do what was best for me to survive and improve my health. This was something that was hard as a teenager but in my current situation was a necessity.

I guess you could say things were moving in the right direction. It was but it still was not as much progress as I had hoped for. I was progressing but at a slower rate than I would have liked. I still was not yet driving. My energy could have been even better. One of the most troubling things was my lack of ability to focus. I was beginning to wonder if I would ever see a day where I did not feel fatigue, shortness of breath, chest pain, and have spouts of rapid heart rate. Plus, none of my results from the orthostatic tests that my school nurse did everyday was changing from the first day of school. I had a couple good days but overall the numbers stayed the same. It usually was a heart rate of between 75-90 when sitting and 130 or higher when standing.

Next was my follow up visit with Dr. Hubbard. I explained how everything was going. He was happy with the progress but we wanted to figure out ways to speed up the process. He took me off the salt tablet since it was not helping much and could be part of the reason for my high blood pressure. One thing he did prescribe me was Vyvanse an ADHD medication. He felt like this would help with my focusing. The medication is designed to send more blood flow to the head. As long as there were no major complications he felt like it could work.

To my surprise, the Vyvanse actually started to help speed up my progress. It did cause some side effects such as cold hands and feet, lack of appetite, sleep disturbances, and most embarrassing of all, I had a hard time getting an erection but it did seem to give me some boost of energy and ability to focus better. As the next couple weeks went by I was progressing to only one trip to the nurse a day. I was feeling up to going to meet with my cross country teammates after school every day and no longer was having to use a stool to sit down to take a shower. I even started driving short distances such as back and forth to school each day. I was extremely pleased with my recent progress. The Vyvanse did not help me feel one hundred percent by any means but it did seem to give me an extra energy boost to push through stuff. My ability to focus improved dramatically as well.

Next up was my visit back to Penn State Hershey Medical Center with Dr. Levine. After talking and discussing issues with her, she and I both agreed the depression medication was not doing much so she decided to take me off it. With my recent progress and being that Hershey was a longer trip for me, she thought I was fine to just be seen by Dr. Hubbard. She was happy with the way everything was going and let me know that if I started going backwards again she was always there for help.

Things were continuing to go up and so was my mood. Come mid November I finally got to the point where I no longer need to stop at the nurse to rest anymore. I continually stopped by to get my orthostatic test results done daily which were continuing to keep slightly improving. I also was increasing my driving distances as well. By no means was I one hundred percent, during my physically therapy sessions I had yet begun to do any running, swimming or heavy physical activity but I had learned to adapt, cope, and survive to live a pretty normal everyday life.

I kept following up with Dr. Hubbard and on my next visit with the progress I was making we decided to take my physical therapy up a notch. Practices for Volleyball were going to start at end of February and practices for winter club volleyball would start in a month. For the next month I really went hard on the aqua and off land physical therapy. We started from a slight jog, to running and mini sprints. We started from one lap of swimming, up to four. I was often exhausted after these workouts but with a healthy diet and the proper rest my body would adjust and slowly progress. I was having no setbacks. I kept dreaming of the day I would be back to one hundred percent. For once it seemed like a real possibility.

A month went by and it was time for club volleyball practices. During the winter our school had a club volleyball team to help prepare us for the spring season.

These were once a week on a Sunday. Dr. Hubbard advised me I could go practice but to start out slow and if I felt it was too much to stop. I was also advised that even though practice was two hours, to start at one hour for my first practice and continue to build myself up to two hours. Again, with staying the course, eating a healthy diet and getting proper amount of rest by mid January I was a full participant in our Sunday practices. I was also a full participant in a tournament if we had one instead of a practice on Sunday.

In the beginning of February, I went back to Dr. Hubbard for a follow up. Everything kept getting better from my orthostatic numbers, to my energy, stamina, and feeling in my limbs. I was happy with the progress but I still did not feel I was at my one hundred percent strength and had regained full ability to focus yet. Tryouts for Volleyball were a little over three weeks away so Dr. Hubbard decided to increase my ADHD medication hoping this would help in getting me closer to full strength.

I started taking a higher dosage of Vyvanse for about a week but apparently this was too much for my body to handle. A week after I increased my dosage I was in 7th period Entrepreneurship class and absolutely felt terrible. It started from the time school started and got worse as the school day proceeded. For medicine that was supposed to increase my focus for some reason at this time I could not focus. I was dizzy, nausea, and had tremendous amount of head pressure. For not having to stop down at the nurse to rest for over two and a half months I had no choice but to go.

Once I got down to the nurse, the nurse was surprised to see me but automatically could tell I did not look good. In fact, I must have looked terrible because she had a slight bit of panic when she was testing me. I lied down and she immediately took my blood pressure. It was an astounding 195/110. I was told by her that I immediately had to go to the hospital with a blood pressure like that. So the nurse contacted my mom and off to the hospital the school transported me.

Once at the hospital they did a bunch of tests. As usual all the tests came back absolutely normal. When asked if I had taken any new medications recently, I informed him no but that my Vyvanse dosage was recently increased. After I told him this the doctor immediately seemed to think this was the problem. My body had a bad reaction to the increased dosage of Vyvanse, which is a stimulant. The increased dosage was too much for my body and caused my blood pressure to sky rocket through the roof. He directed me to go back to the original dosage and to follow up with Dr. Hubbard.

I followed up with Dr. Hubbard and we talked about my issue with the increase dosage. Besides going back to the original dose he thought at this point with what had happened, to stop the Vyvanse for good and see how my body does without it. I agreed. I was a little nervous since the Vyvanse seemed to help a little but it did give me side effects such as loss of appetite, constant cold hands and feet, erectile dysfunction but these are symptoms that I just began to cope with. Despite the positives, the negatives at the time outweighed the positives from my use of Vyvanse, hence, it was discontinued.

I was a little nervous now if I was going to recover enough to be cleared to play volleyball which had been my goal all school year. I was practicing and playing once a week but there is a big difference between once a week and when Spring season starts. During spring season, Volleyball would then be five days a week.

I was just taken off Vyvanse and I had not felt well since the day I recently ended up in the hospital. I was hoping the original increase in Vyvanse would not do anything to give me a set back with my P.O.T.S. I was eager to think that now; once it got out of my system it would blow over. That I would return to how I was feeling before the increase in dosage. I only had two weeks until my follow up physical with Dr. Hubbard. This physical was to determine if I was healthy enough to be a full go participant at volleyball tryouts for the upcoming season. Since, being a senior I already knew I would make the team.

The day arrived for my physical with Dr. Hubbard and a decision was to be made. Luckily, the hospital incident did not set me back and once the Vyvanse left my system I seemed to go back to where I was previously. I was feeling good. I was not one hundred percent back to my old self like I was the year before. I realized that but I just hoped I would be deemed healthy enough to play. Dr. Hubbard requested that I brought the results of the readings the school nurse was recording for me daily along with me so he could go over the results to help him make a final decision. He looked over the results and we talked about how I had been feeling since being taken off the Vyvanse. Fortunately, I had seen no negative change in my health since being taken off the drug. He did the normal physical checkup and came to the decision that I would be healthy enough to play volleyball the upcoming season. He told me by the look of my results all my numbers with my heart rate and blood pressure were getting back to normal and that my tests showed no signs of tachycardia from sitting down to standing up within the past two weeks. We also left it off that I would not need to have any more follow up visits unless I started feeling really ill again.

I was extremely excited to hear this news. To think of where I had come from since the first day I was diagnosed with P.O.T.S. completely blew my mind. All the doctors and nurses I encountered were impressed as well. I started to believe that it was only a matter of time until I was back to the one hundred percent old self. If I was healthy enough to play a high school sport again than it should only be a matter of time.

Adjusting to My New Life

The first week of volleyball practices were rough. I was still not in shape but after a week I began to adjust. My cardio kept improving but eventually it stalled. After a month or so I realized that I still was not one hundred percent. I would still get dizzy, off balance at times and never fully regained complete spatial sensation back. Due to this I was able to compete but not at the highest level that I used to for the volleyball season.

Realizing I was not going to be as athletic and good at sports as I once was became disappointing but after everything I went through I was just happy to be able to participate in sports again and feel like a normal seventeen-year-old human being. The jury was still out on if I was going to ever fully recover from Postural Orthostatic Tachycardia Syndrome. I heard multiple answers from doctors. Some said you could and others stated you never will. I was beginning to be under the impression that I never would. Frustrating at times but it was something I would have to adjust to. The one thing that kept me happy was I knew I already made progress from where I used to be and I could still function like an everyday citizen with not many limitations.

Being able to finish the volleyball season with no issues was a very satisfying feeling and one I viewed as a huge accomplishment. The upcoming summer I was a lifeguard at the Antietam Pool and did not have to call off from work for any health issues. It felt good to not feel as if I was being viewed as weak or crazy again. It was not always easy but I made adjustments to cope with my P.O.T.S. symptoms to make it through the day. My body would not be able to handle the heat as well but one thing I did to help with this is constantly have an umbrella above my lifeguarding chair, as well as take multiple dips in the pool throughout the day. Driving was another everyday norm I could do again with no distance restrictions. During long drives at times I would get a racing heart, sweaty hands or light headedness but I was at the point my body could now push through it without passing out. It may not have been safe. There were plenty of times I should have pulled over to stop but I never did. During these long drives these symptoms would occur but I would just push through it. The symptoms would last anywhere from a half hour to an hour but eventually would go away. It could be scary at times especially for the passengers with me but one thing that helped was that I believed it was not going to kill me and I would constantly ensure my passengers that I was fine.

Next step was college. This was going to be a big step. I was going to Indiana University of Pennsylvania (IUP); a state school located an hour northwest of Pittsburgh and a very big party school. Some say the IUP stood for" I Usually Party." Not only that but I was going to be all on my own. It was going to be interesting to see how my health would hold up.

To make the transition easier my family and I notified the health center on campus of my medical condition and had appointments set up with a neurologist to keep up with my health. The RA was notified of my health and they put my dorm room right across from his.

College from a health standpoint turned-out better than expected. During the course of my four years I went on my share of doctors' appointments. I had a couple scares. I ended up in the emergency room four times during my four years at IUP. Overall, I found some positive and negatives in how the college lifestyle affected my P.O.T.S.

The positive was all the walking I did from class, to social events and parties. I worked out at the gym sporadically but all the walking really helped improve my cardio. Most college students gain the freshman fifteen but with my metabolism that did not happen and with all the walking I did my cardiovascular health seemed better than it did when I was at home on breaks I was surrounded by tons of friends. Even if I was having a bad day I was surrounded by many people that could make me laugh or constantly having me involved in something fun that would keep my mind off things. The last positive thing was if I really did feel horrible I could sleep and rest as much as I wanted to recover. I could move at my own pace. School was no longer a mandatory thing to attend. If I did not feel well I just would not go to class and get the notes from someone else in my class.

For all the positives there were two negatives. One was if I was having issues no one there knew what was wrong with me. Having postural orthostatic tachycardia syndrome was something I never mentioned to people I met either. It is so hard to comprehend and I did not want people to judge me as being the sick or weak guy. I did not want to miss out on making friends because of a bizarre illness I was unfortunate enough to be diagnosed with. I wanted everyone to think I was just like them. In moments where my P.O.T.S. symptoms would flare up I found myself making excuses like I was just dehydrated or had a cold. The last negative was drinking. Just like 90 percent of all college students, I drank and partied. I was always a competitive person and I brought this mentality with me when it came to college partying. I did not want anyone to outdrink me or think I was not a man because I could not handle my liquor. Due to this I did build up quite the tolerance. Surprisingly, during my college years the excessive drinking never caused a huge relapse with my

P.O.T.S.Where the P.O.T.S. did make a difference was in recovering from hangovers after a weekend or rough night of drinking. As most other young college people could still function their everyday life with a hangover it was extremely difficult for me. I would get chest pains, it would flare up symptoms. I would often sleep all day and my day consisted of nothing but resting. I did not even have the energy do to any school work most times. I could drink just as much as your average frat star during the night or weekend but I sure could not recover like one. Recoveries took much longer than a day for me.

Once I came home from college I got a job at a bank as a part-time teller. While I was home I went to work every day normally. In fact, at one point I even worked two jobs. One as a teller and one as a sales associate at the Boscov's Department Store for seasonal help. I was feeling better than I ever had. A lot of times I would even forget that I was suffering from Postural Orthostatic Tachycardia Syndrome. In fact, there was only two times I ever felt symptoms flare up. One was after a usual night of too much drinking and the second was when working out at the gym. When working out at the gym and playing sports, I usually went with one of my best friends, Kyle Sheetz. We lived real close to one another and played on the men's volleyball team together in high school; during our workouts he was also able to push himself a lot harder than me. After a certain amount of time I would get dizzy, lightheaded, and a racing heart. I would have to stop my workout or bring the intensity down. During the summer, I participated on a slow pitch softball team. I was one of the best hitters on the team but running around the bases or in the outfield was usually a challenge. Some of my friends would be amazed at how out of breath I could get at times. I was more out of breath than my teammates who constantly smoked cigarettes or whose diet was not as healthy as mine.

Despite not being able to push myself physically as much as I would like or maybe as the model average athlete could, I was still happy with my life. I lived like a normal person and still could accomplish all my career goals and dreams. I had not had a huge relapse in my symptoms that made me as sick as I was when I was first diagnosed at seventeen-years-old. I was content with this fact and figured this would be how I would feel for the rest of my life. It seemed as if my P.OT.S. had plateaued or so I thought. Little did I know I would be in for a huge surprise.

Relapses

One thing I never mentioned in the previous chapter is that when I left IUP I hit some hard times. I was allowed to walk at graduation but I still had two classes to finish up. I told my advisor I would finish them up that summer so I could still walk. I was scheduled to be done in four years but unfortunately, I did not always make the right choices. My whole life I have been a competitive person. I like the feeling of being "The Man" as they would say. Even though I was never in a frat, this mindset led me to live the frat star lifestyle during my four years at IUP. Instead of being competitive in out-studying and out-working everyone, I was competitive in trying to out-drink and out-party everyone. The consequences of this were I failed a couple classes and would not be able to complete all my college credits necessary to graduate within four years as planned.

Besides being ultra-competitive, I also had lots of pride. One thing I hated most was seeing my mother and father disappointed in me. So needless to say, I tried to keep the fact that I still needed to finish two classes (I failed) to receive my diploma a secret.

This secret only lasted so long, midway through the summer a notice came in the mail I still needed more credits to graduate. I tried to play it off at first that it was not my fault and that my advisor must have made a mistake. Instead of being honest I tried to make it seem as if my professor miscalculated my credits and because of him I have to take one more class this summer.

I did indeed take one class that summer but again I failed it. Scared to let my parents know I failed I told them everything was all good and I would eventually get my diploma. I thought that I could keep just buying myself time until I finally finished those two classes online.

The secret that I had not finished all credits to graduate was not the only thing that was bothering me and going on in my life. Not being in college anymore was an adjustment. The real world is nothing like being on a college campus. Living in a world that I had to be a complete adult was not fun to me yet, and to know some of my friends were having fun at back at college was depressing. I was completely unhappy in the real world which caused me to have a real piss poor attitude. I could not seem to face reality that it was time to grow up. I hated everything about the real world at this time. Life was not just about how fun you were, adventurous you could be, or how you liked to party. You no longer lived in a house with your best friends going through life without a care in the world. You were no longer just judged on your sense of humor or personality because everyone around you was in the same boat. No the real world was different. You seemed to be judged on how successful you were, how much knowledge you had, and whole bunch of other intangibles you could bring to the table. I like to say I was not ready for the real world yet, but looking back I just needed a new shift in mindset and a different attitude.

The thing that really messed up with my head is what happened next. During my last year at IUP I started dating this woman from the Delta Phi Epsilon sorority in the very beginning of the first semester. She lived in the complex above me. Which if you saw how it was laid out; you could basically say we lived in the same house. We dated the whole school year. We did not have the best relationship. We had our good and bad moments. Once school was over our relationship changed. Being away from the IUP atmosphere had done our relationship good. We were becoming closer than ever. It was almost approaching a year and I will admit I was slowly becoming in love with this woman at the time.

Unfortunately, times were going to start getting tougher again in our relationship. Unlike me, she had to go back to IUP for one more year. We were going to be four hours apart now living completely different lifestyles. I was determined to make it work and I hoped she was too. The distance began to take its toll within the first month and I could tell things were not going well. I did not want to let go though. I had already made up my mind at that time that this was the woman I wanted to be with for the rest of my life. I believed if we could just make it through the school year everything would be fine. That did not happen. Third week of September, as we were almost at a year in, she broke up with me with no explanation except that she need time away from everything. She blamed it on that she was not happy anymore. Insisting that she had personal issues she needed to take care of. Later, I found out the real reason. She had been cheating on me with some other guy she began dating. He was a twenty-seven-year-old doctorate student at the time. Not only this, but they were officially dating before we even broke up. This is confirmed by both of their Facebook statuses to this day. It shows they have been in a relationship since August 26th; we did not officially break up until September 21st.

The breakup hit me extremely hard and set me into a complete depression. I am embarrassed to admit it but I even considered suicide a couple times. For someone that took so much pride in "Feeling like the Man". I was weak all together. I was weak in all three phases again: mentally, physically, and emotionally. Just how I was when I was first diagnosed with P.O.T.S. when I was seventeen. The only difference was this time it was not completely caused by P.O.T.S. It was a combination of P.O.T.S. and a whole bunch of external factors. I felt like a huge disappointment to my family for not finishing my degree on time and was having anxiety over them not knowing the truth. I felt like I did not fit in with the real world quite yet and was miserable. Now I was wondering why all the sudden out of nowhere I was not good enough for the woman I loved and did everything for at the time.

With everything coming down on me at once I felt I had to get at least one thing off my chest so I finally decided to tell my mom and dad the news that I still had not finished my degree and had two more classes to go. Needless to say, they were both extremely disappointed and upset with me. They both informed me I was on my own now and I was going to have to figure out a way to finish the classes, pay for everything and suffer the consequences. I had no problem with this. I realized I had no one else to blame but myself.

My mom took the news of me not finishing my classes to graduate harder than my father did. I could tell it really hurt her and upset her, rightfully so. She would let her frustrations out on me from time to time trying to talk to me about how I could be so irresponsible and let this happen and lie to her. She had a point and I had no one else to blame but with everything else that was going on and being depressed I did not want to hear it. We got in an argument and this time I decided to leave. I packed up all my bags and moved in with my dad. I was in a horrible state of mind and wanted to try and get away from everyone I disappointed and just wanted time to figure myself out. I realized I was incredibly depressed and did not have my life together. I wanted to try and get back to being happy again and get my head on straight. For some reason at this time I thought getting away from everyone and everything would make that happen.

I went the whole next year until November without talking to my mother. During this time, I was a complete wreck. I went to work every day but I drank every single weekend, and heavily. I might have not been in college anymore but I kept drinking like I was still in my college days. It got so bad that one night I had to be carried into my house by one of my friends because I was blacked out unconscious. I do not remember anything but I woke to puke all over my clothes, bed, bedroom and bathroom floors. This even set my dad off. My dad, who usually is not that hard on me, then threatened that if I ever came home like that again that I needed to find a new place to stay. The only good thing I did during this time was finish my classes so I could finally receive my Bachelor's degree that summer. The only thing was I did not have any money to get my diploma, since I could not pay off my tuition. I was currently just working as a landscaper and all the money I did make I was blowing on going out and partying every weekend.

Still not accepting the fact that I was not a college student anymore, late October I decided to reconnect with some old IUP friends. We decided to make a trip up to Penn State to visit their one friend who was a senior at Penn State at the time. We were going up to see a primetime football game that was to be aired at 8pm on ABC. This football game was going to be as Penn State calls it a "Whiteout" because all 100,000 plus fans in the stadium wear white. The game was against Ohio State one of the top teams in the country at the time. Again, I want insane. I drank and drank some more. We got there late Friday afternoon and did not stop drinking until early Monday morning when I had gotten kicked out of a bar for being too intoxicated. I had been drinking alcohol for literally three days straight.

I woke up later Monday morning and I felt terrible. I usually always felt horrible after a weekend of drinking but something felt different. Twenty minutes after we hopped in my friend's car on the ride home everything seemed to go bonkers. I literally could not feel anything, I was dizzy, I felt like I was going to pass out and my heart was flying faster than ever. I usually pull it together when I was around my friends but I was so scared I caused a scene. After so many years of not having this feeling like I was dying, I had it again. My friends looked up the closest hospital and took me to one. They were concerned but were not sure as to what made me act so crazy. Never in their life had they seen me act like that. To them I was just a normal athletic twenty-three -year old.

At the Lewisburg Hospital, they put me in the emergency room and did a bunch of tests. They could not find anything wrong. They acknowledged my blood pressure was tremendously high and my heart rate was too but no tests showed anything serious. The doctor told me that I was just extremely dehydrated (which tests did prove) and that I was just to drink plenty of fluids, get solid rest, and I would be okay. All I did was rest on the way home and prayed the doctor was right. This feeling was oh too familiar but I did not want to think the worst just yet. Not only that but I was embarrassed how I just acted in front my friends. I just wanted to get home and sleep. Hoping I would wake up the next day and everything would be all right.

I woke up the next day and did not feel better one bit at all. I figured I did a lot of damage to my body over the weekend so I just need a full day to eat, drink healthy and get plenty of rest. That is exactly what I did all day. I do not recall even moving from the couch. I went to bed at 8pm since I had to be up at 6:30am for work. I woke up at 6:30am but I still did not feel right. In fact, I felt worse than

I had the previous day before. All the rest did nothing. I tried to push myself to get ready and hoped if I made it to work I would be fine. I would never make it that far. As I walked outside to my car I got extremely dizzy and felt like I was almost going to pass out. I laid down and called my boss and told him I was not feeling well and I would not be able to make it in to work.

I was petrified. I was dizzy, my heart was flying, I lost feeling in my limbs again. I knew something was wrong. Unlike in the past, the day of rest and healthy eating did nothing. I felt as If I was getting worse by the day. This made me begin to think the worst was happening fast. I was convicned I wanted to go to the hospital. I was sure during my last trip to the Lewisburg Hospital on the way home from Penn State they must have missed something. There is no way if everything was perfectly okay with me I would still be feeling like this. I ended up calling my father at work. He agreed to leave work to come home and take me to the hospital.

On my way to the hospital I literally felt like I was dying. As if my heart was going to beat out my chest or I was just going to wither away. I was extremely fatigued and weak. I could not even walk by myself and as soon as we hit the emergency room I was placed in a wheelchair right away as I almost collapsed getting out my dad's truck. They immediately rushed me back into a room and started doing tests.

Besides my blood pressure being very high along with my heart rate all the tests for my heart came back normal. Eventually, after sitting awhile my heart rate started to decline as well. The doctors were very disturbed by what they saw when I first arrived so they decided to have me spend the night and get more tests and a cat scan done. Once I woke up in the morning and the doctor got all the results he informed me that all the tests came back and that everything was normal. He did notice I had a history of P.O.T.S. and wanted to do a tilt table test on me. Once he did the tilt table test, the doctor had no doubt in his mind that the P.O.T.S. symptoms had come back and increased with a vengeance. My heart rate nearly doubled from sitting to standing. He informed me this could be due to the overly excessive drinking I had done over the weekend and that with P.O.T.S. I cannot continue this behavior or things like this are going to continue to happen. He made it very clear that being an excessive drinker could lead to worse case scenarios that I did not want to think about or other people may never experience.

For the next week when I got home I was severely depressed. Here I was back at the same stage when I was seventeen-years-old, which had now been six years ago, in regards to my P.O.T.S. symptoms. All I kept thinking was how long it took me to fully recover that I could live a so called normal life again. Last time it took me six months to get my life back to normalcy and that was when I was younger. Even then six months was beating the odds. Not only that but now I was going to be out of work for a while. I really felt like a loser more now than ever. I ran away from my mom, step dad, sister and brother hoping to find happiness again but here I was even more depressed. I finally finished all my credits to graduate from IUP but now I had no job to even try to make money to pay off my tuition to receive my diploma or have my college submit transcripts to future employers. I was broke, not even healthy enough to drive at the time being, and had no job. I was trying to find another female companion to help take away the pain I had at the time of my ex-girlfriend leaving and cheating on me but who the heck would want me now. I had nothing going for me. Again, I was 23, still living at home, had no job, completely broke, can barely do anything because of my health, and have been running away from all the people that did care about me.

I'll admit after a week went by, one night I was falling asleep crying but then something out nowhere hit me. Just like every time in the past I was having a moment thinking deeply and trying to fall asleep. I realized what is crying going to do? I realized I needed to swallow my pride and look in the mirror. The truth was at that exact moment I was a loser. I had to accept that fact. I also realized that I *did not* have to be a loser forever. My actions are the ones that put me in the situation I was in but if I could change my actions I could change the situation I was currently in. I also admitted to myself I needed help. I was depressed. Everyone could tell and everyone knew it. It was to the point I needed help. I did not like the thought of having to talk to a psychiatrist but I knew it was what was best for me. I also realized I needed to apologize to my mother, step dad, brother and sister and be part of the family again. They were right. I was wrong. By running away, I thought I could run away from my problems but all it did was make them worse. Last but not least, I needed to calm down on the partying and drinking. I was not only doing this for my health but also to help me financially, mentally and emotionally. I realized the reason I drank so much was because it was like I was only happy when I was drunk. I tried to drink away my problems. Besides drinking to be happy I also thought going out every weekend and try having random hook ups would take away the pain of my breakup. Everything I was doing was wrong. It was just sending me into a downward spiral.

The next morning, I woke up with a new attitude. I explained to my dad how I thought I needed to see someone and he agreed and set me up with an appointment with a psychiatrist. I also texted my mom and sent her a long apology and let her know I wanted to be part of the family's life again. Next, I realized I needed to stop focusing on women and partying and focus on bettering me. Last but not least I needed to set myself up on some program to help me recover from P.O.T.S., which I did.

The next three months were some of the most life changing months in my life. I went to a psychiatrist weekly and it felt good to talk to someone. I was prescribed Cymbalta depression medication. Besides hearing horror stories from other people, I responded well to this medication.

As for my mom, she responded to my apology and I met up with the family. I apologized and I started getting more involved. It felt good to see and be part of the family. I also worked extremely hard on myself. I did not drink at all for all those three months. I learned to have fun without alcohol. I had great support from my closest friends. Most of them lived close by and understood I could not drive yet due to my P.O.T.S. They picked me up almost every day to hangout. They were also supportive in my non-drinking. At nights, we normally would have gone out, we now stayed in and would play videogames, watch movies, or YouTube videos, even when we would go out they never pressured me to drink. They respected the new me. I explained to them that even when I was healthier I was going to cut down on the drinking and partying. I explained the only time I would drink is when I had accomplished something and a reason to celebrate. Even then I would monitor myself and not get out of control. In fact, I have no desire to ever get drunk again to be honest.

The physical therapy, healthy diet, and proper rest really helped my P.O.T.S. start to go in remission. A little after three months since I had my hospital visit in the beginning of February 2015, I started driving again. I was starting to feel happier than I had ever been. I was motivated; I restored the relationship with my mother, step dad, brother, and sister. I cut back tremendously on the alcohol and partying, and I was physically able to live a so called normal life again. I finally felt it was time to start applying for jobs.

After just a week of applying I heard back from a job I applied for with the Hertz Corporation. It was to be a manager trainee at the branch in my hometown of Reading, Pennsylvania with the goal to keep moving up. I went for the interview and everything went great. I got a call back a couple days later and they offered me the position and I was scheduled to start in two weeks. All I had to do was pass a drug test and have IUP send my transcripts over.

I was ecstatic to get offered the job but I was nervous about my transcripts because IUP told me they could not send any until I paid off my tuition. I had no choice so I decided to call IUP and beg to give me an exception. They told me they would honor to send my transcripts as a one-time only thing if I agreed to put some money down and continue to pay on it. All I had was sixty-six dollars in my account. I told them the most I could put down was fifty dollars as that was all I really had. The secretary for the billing office at IUP did not seem too happy with that and said she would have to speak with her manager. After speaking with the manager, however, they allowed for me to pay fifty dollars down and they would send my transcripts under the agreement that I would continue to pay on it or they would send it to collections. I agreed and it felt like a world was lifted off my shoulders. I only was going to have sixteen bucks to my name but I was about to start making money soon. I finally had a job that required a college degree and was going to pay me a decent wage.

I started my new job and everything was going great. I was determined to make a good impression and work my way up quick. In fact, as soon as August I was promoted to manager associate. I was really good at what I did. I could sell, I had a strong business mindset, and last but not least I was working my ass off. If they needed me to I would work close to sixty hours if I could. Heck, sometimes just to make a good impression I would stay late and work extra hours even when it was not required.

Everything was going well. I continued my way of continuing to work out, ate healthy, and rarely drank or partied. Financially I was doing well too. I was no longer blowing my money on alcohol and even paid off all my tuition and received my degree in the mail. I even got a new girlfriend in November. Her name is Maddie Barbitta. She is beautiful and I could tell she liked me a lot. She was very patient with me and understanding of my P.O.T.S. I was happy about this. I was already happy with how everything was going and she just made me happier. She became the new love of my life.

In February, just a little under a year from when I started at Hertz I was promoted to assistant branch manager. Just around the same time my friends and I planned a trip to Mardi Gras. Yes I drank but I did not drink more than one day in a row. I was proud of myself.

When I came back from the trip I could not wait to keep moving my way up. Next promotion would be to Branch Manager which came with special perks such as a gas card and company car. I continued to work really hard. Around May my normal slow pitch softball season began. During softball season, I could not quite work as many hours as I usually would, especially this season since I was going to be hosting a charity softball tournament in August with all proceeds going to Four Diamonds of Penn State Medical Center.

Despite being super busy and stressed out I was feeling good. I did not need to see a psychiatrist or physical therapist since I started at Hertz which had been over a year. I figured the healthiest option was to be medication free and do everything naturally. So, in July, I took a trip to the doctor and we figured out a plan to wean me off my depression medication. I heard horror stories from people trying to wean off Cymbalta but I figured under Doctor's care, I should be alright. We started out lowering my dose by twenty milligrams and then taking it once every other day for two weeks until I would be completely off. Weaning me off the medication seemed fine or at least I thought so.

Around mid August I kept getting a stuffy nose that I only could get rid of with nasal spray. I went to the doctor and they told me I had an infection and prescribed me antibiotics. The antibiotics did not do anything at all. So, a week later I went back. This time the doctor prescribed me a steroid to clear up my system. The steroid worked wonders, it cleared my system up all right but the side effects were horrible. The steroids kept causing me to cramp up and have terrible pains in my legs. I went to the doctor because of this and they took blood tests and determined my potassium was extremely low. Luckily, it was my last day of taking the steroid. After a week of being off the steroid my potassium levels were normal again but I still was not feeling right. I thought maybe with so much unsureness and difficulties I went through just to clear up a stuffy nose that it could just be anxiety and to push through it,

A couple days later I woke up in the middle of the night, again to go pee just as I did when I was seventeen-years-old. As I started to pee, my heart started racing out of nowhere. I kept hoping unlike when I was seventeen I would not start to black out. When I finished urinating I quickly hopped in my bed and lied down and tried to relax. My heart rate was not going down though and I even told my girlfriend that I was scared. She asked if I wanted to go to the hospital. I told her "No" and that "Hopefully if I fall asleep I will wake up and everything will be okay". I eventually fell asleep. When I woke up my heart was not racing anymore but I felt absolutely terrible. I had a hard time concentrating and I was nauseous. I kept telling myself it had to be anxiety and to push through it. I went to work and I tried to eat lunch but I could not. I was too sick to my stomach. After lunch, it was my duty to go on a couple sales calls to body shops and State Farm agents to draw up and bring in more business. As I left the one State Farm agent's office about twenty-five minutes from our office in Reading I was feeling so horrible that I was afraid to drive back. I did not know what could possibly be wrong with me, so like always I kept telling myself it is just anxiety and I drove off. Five minutes into driving my heart started racing again and it was only getting worse. I knew I needed to pull over. I saw a body shop on the side of the road and thought it would be perfect. I pulled over and told myself maybe if I walk to get some fresh air and start talking to people to get my mind off my body I would feel better. I walked into the body shop and the first thing the lady asked if I was okay. I told her "Yeah I am fine." Little did I know those would be the last words I would say to her.

Next thing I knew, I woke up and I was being pulled into an ambulance. I was told that I had just blacked out. Now I was really scared. I had never completely blacked out and awakened in an ambulance before. They took me to the hospital and did tons of tests. After about six hours after performing a bunch of tests they could not figure out what was wrong. They doctor told me it was most likely a withdrawal reaction from not taking the Cymbalta anymore and they decided to put me back on the medication. He also believed I was not handling all the stress well and thought I was having a bad anxiety. He also prescribed me Ativan, an anxiety medication.

I took a couple medical days off and then decided to take a week off from work. During my week off I also got exciting news. The branch manager who used to work at the Norristown location fifty minutes from Reading was moving on and they were going to promote me to Branch Manager when I returned back to work. I was so excited. It seemed all my hard work was paying off. Now all I had to do was get healthy. I figured being put back on the medication would change things.

A week went by and it was time to go back to work. I did not feel much better but today was a huge day and I could not call off. I went to work and after an hour of handing my stuff in, it was time to drive down to Norristown to get my big promotion. I was excited. I was thinking how cool it was going to be to never have to drive my personal car nor pay for gas again. Fifteen minutes into the drive my excitement went away. All I was doing was driving and relaxing, in a good mood since I was getting promoted but my heart kept racing faster and faster. I had lost of feeling in my limbs, dizzy and it felt like I was going to blackout any second. I had no choice but to pull over. It finally dawned on me that I was not experiencing withdrawal or anxiety symptoms anymore. I was back on Cymbalta and totally sedated on high doses of Ativan but yet I was still having these symptoms. I was all too familiar with this feeling.

I picked up my cell phone and called my dad and told him I needed to be picked up and taken home, that it was not safe for me to drive. He realized that something was wrong and he did indeed pick me up. Once he picked me up he was asked what was going on. I told him right away that my P.O.T.S. is back. I do not know why but I feel the exact way I did when I was seventeen and two years ago, after my wild weekend at Penn State.

We made an appointment with a doctor and he confirmed after doing the tilt table test that I indeed was suffering from increased P.O.T.S. Symptoms. My heart rate when lying down was 64. When standing up it was 151. He did not know when I could return to work but I was going to have to take it easy and focus on recovering again. Unlike last time when the cause of relapse was alcohol poisoning the doctor had no answer for the relapse in symptoms this time. Only thing he could come up with was too much stress, possibly the withdrawal I originally suffered from being taken off Cymbalta, or the side effects of the steroid I had taken. No one honestly knew what caused my relapse this time. It just happened.

I did not know how to feel when I got home. I called my boss and disappointedly told him I would have to decline the promotion as I needed to focus on my health to get better. As for how long I would be out of work I did not know. It would be longer than all my vacation days so I had two options. I could file for medical leave or I could leave the company. I told him I needed time to think about it. I needed time to think about a lot of things. It felt like every time I made progress in my life that my P.O.T.S. would always set me back. In fact, it was like the only thing holding me back. I was tired of living like this. I needed time to think, clear my mind, and figure out how I was going to cope with this bizarre syndrome. A syndrome that once I felt I beat would come back out of nowhere, a syndrome that was affecting my life tremendously, and a syndrome that so many people seemed to not understand. I was making all the right decisions in my life and I still could not get rid of this thing called Postural Orthostatic Tachycardia Syndrome. This thing was ruining my life.

Other P.O.T.S. Stories

Now that you heard my story, I would like to share others' stories that have been diagnosed with P.O.T.S. You have learned my story, how P.O.T.S has affected my life and the loved ones around me. I want to bring awareness to Postural Orthostatic Tachycardia Syndrome and I knew in order to do this it was going to take more than just my story. As I was taught as a young kid playing sports, "Big teams accomplish big dreams" and I believe that with all my heart to this day. I wanted to interview other people with P.O.T.S. so you can see not how P.O.T.S has just affected mine but also many other people's lives as well.

Being such an unknown disease I wanted to try and find as many people that were going through what I was going through. I was not sure how successful I would be when first started. I knew there were almost one million people diagnosed but again P.O.T.S is not something you hear of very often. Luckily, with tons of googling, YouTube and social media searches, (especially the Postural Orthostatic Tachycardia Syndrome Group on Facebook) I was able to find some. In fact, I was able to find interviews with people of all genders, ages, and different parts of the world. None of that would have been possible if it was not for social media. It is incredible how social media can connect us with people all over the world. It got to the point where I actually was unable to share everyone's story that wanted to, but I did the best I could.

As I began to share with everyone my idea of creating a book, I was encouraged by all the support, I could tell the impact P.O.T.S had on all these people. Everyone was thrilled to find someone that wanted to bring awareness to something that they have been struggling with and wanted to help even if it meant sharing their personal story (though I removed all last names to keep their privacy). While reading all the interviews I would encourage you to read all of them carefully. Everyone has their own story and each is just as important as the rest. Take a look at some of the similarities and the wide array of symptoms and effects this syndrome has had on people. During some of the interviews you will hear the people refer to a group called "Potsies". This is sometimes what people suffering with P.O.T.S refer to other P.O.T.S patients as. You will begin to see the big need for awareness and attention to be brought to Postural Orthostatic Tachycardia Syndrome. Here are my interviews. Here are their stories.

Connor, 21 Years Old

1.) First tell me a little bit about yourself? (Name, age, hobbies, anything interesting)

Connor. I'm currently 22 years old. I am also Canadian, so possibly my process has been different than that of an American. My hobbies used to include working on cars, hanging out with friends, driving, and occasionally playing sports just for fun. Since August 2015 my life has been very different and even the small amount of hobbies I used to enjoy I no longer can.

2.) When were you first diagnosed with P.O.T.S.?

I was diagnosed with POTS and ME/CFS on the same day, June 6th 2016. Shortly after I was diagnosed with Fibromyalgia as well.

3.) How long did the process take? How many doctors did you have to see until you finally got an official diagnosis?

My first day off work without returning, eventually leading to being laid off, was August 31st 2015. I was originally misdiagnosed with Pneumonia and given antibiotics for months. I was then sent by my family GP to a lung specialist. She performed several lung tests and referred me to get an Echo-cardiogram through another heart specialist. This test then came back with results that were misinterpreted as me having a Ventricular Septal Defect, (VSD) the believed seriousness at the time had those 2 specialists conclude I needed to be sent to Pacific Adult Congenital Heart Clinic where I was then referred. The PACH Clinic then found different results to that of the previous heart specialist and I was cleared of a VSD. Shortly after being referred to the PACH Clinic I had also been referred to the Rapid Access Clinic to see the doctor that eventually diagnosed me. My first appointment with the RA Clinic was with a student doctor who sent me for every kind of blood, spit, and fluid test possible. I returned to the RA Clinic months later, June 6th 2016, and was finally heard by my current doctor. He was the first doctor that heard all of my symptoms and actually understood what I was talking about. He had me lay down while we continued talking, I had no idea at the time but he was about to diagnose me with POTS. Once 10 minutes of laying down he tested my heart rate which was at 64, asked me to stand up and within 10 second it went to 116. Immediately he knew I had POTS and throughout the rest of the conversation he determined ME/CFS as well. My process took at least 7 doctors, most of which specialists, and from August 29th 2015 until June 6th 2016 to actually get a diagnosis.

4.) When did you first start noticing something was wrong? First symptom or situation?

March 2015, my lungs first starting giving me a hard time. Taking deep breaths is still impossible to today and the issue has not been diagnosed. After this problem in March the onset of other problems followed.

5.) Though most causes are unknown do you have any idea what might have triggered the onset of P.O.T.S.?

The only thing I could say would be the viral infection I had in March 2015. ME/CFS can apparently be brought on by viral or bacterial infections, and my symptoms of POTS and ME/CFS showed up very close to each other in August 2015.

6.) How many trips do you take to a hospital or doctor's office per month? Per year?

I see my family GP every 2-3 weeks. I see my RA Clinic doctor once every 2-3 months specifically for POTS and ME/CFS. Per year unfortunately I can't answer with any kind of accuracy.

7.) Do you believe you will ever fully recover from P.O.T.S. and never have any setbacks?

I do very much so hope to fully recover. Although my issue at the moment is simply the treatment options I have been offered.

8.) How has this syndrome affected your work, school, relationships, and friendships? (Life in general)

I haven't been able to work since August 2015. I was very interested in cars, working for an automotive parts company, and looking into post-secondary schooling to become a mechanic or auto body repairman. Both options for schooling are no longer something I can physically take on, and career wise most likely not options fit for my physical state anymore. Unfortunately. I am only 22 and the majority of my friends and interested in things my body just does not allow. My friendships have definitely changed and been affected by all of this.

9.) What are the worst symptoms you have ever experienced caused by P.O.T.S.?

Blacking out completely. Has thankfully only happened once, following a blood test. After about 30 seconds of being blacked out I woke up and vomited. Again thankfully I was in a lab and had nurses all around me. On a daily basis I deal with lightheadedness, fast heartbeat, spotty vision and occasionally when I stand up total loss of vision for a short period of time but I have never blacked out completely and fallen over at home.

10.) What has helped you recover the best? (Exercise, food diet, attitude)

I have yet to find that. I'm very grateful for my family and my doctors though, their support means the most.

11.) What medications have you been put on to help with P.O.T.S.? Which ones worked and which ones did not?

Originally salt, if that's a medication. Was told to add tons to my food and take heaping spoonfuls several

*times a day. That only worked to produce vomit. I tried
making my own salt tablets, same result. Not sure why my
stomach has such an issue with salt but it really disagrees
with my body: Next was Trazodone, was prescribed for
sleep by RA clinic doctor, family GP asked me not to take
it. Then I was prescribed Amitriptyline also by RA clinic
doc. It was also prescribed for sleep and nerve pain caused
by Fibromyalgia. My family GP does want me to start this
but I haven't done so yet. At the same time I was prescribed
Amitriptyline I was also prescribed Propranolol. My family
GP did not like that RA clinic doctor had prescribed me
this and asked I only do one, she wants Amitriptyline. Salt
unfortunately, like I said before did not work for me. If I
was to change my diet and manage to find a way to work it
in without feeling worse I absolutely would. My eating
habits have been so affected over the last year salt just does
not fit in anywhere. I guess to answer which ones worked, I
haven't tried them. Pharmaceutical drugs honestly scare
me to the point that living with my symptoms is the option I
would rather choose then to take pills every day. I would
love to speak to a Naturopathic doctor and see if there are
options that are natural but they are not covered by
Canadian Health Care and I cannot afford to see one on
my own.*

**12.) Has the P.O.T.S. disease ever caused you to be
depressed or feel like an outcast at any point?**

*I have suffered from depression since early 2013.
My feelings of depression haven't changed because of
POTS. Meaning they haven't gotten better or worse in any
way that I have noticed. Although the difference before
August 2015 and now is that the depression is not the only
thing causing problems. I have felt like an outcast because
of POTS simply because I can't do the same things
everyone else can. I have also tried explaining it to people*

and gotten very weird responses which make me want to not explain it and outcast myself more.

13.) To all those dealing with P.O.T.S. what is the best advice you would give them to cope with everything that this syndrome comes with?

Sorry I really don't know how to answer this.

14.) Do you think there needs to be more awareness brought worldwide in regards to Postural Orthostatic Tachycardia Syndrome?

Absolutely. When I was first diagnosed, I tried to find online communities for both the things I had been diagnosed with and struggled to find anything that had daily activity of people talking about either. POTS and ME/CFS have zero awareness around them and it is definitely an issue. This month has actually been an awareness month for dysautonomia and the exposure it receives is absolutely not comparable to other conditions/syndromes.

Taylor, 21 Years Old

1.) First tell me a little bit about yourself? Name, age, hobbies, anything interesting)

Taylor, 21. I love going to the dog park with my bulldogs and playing piano.

2.) When you were first diagnosed with P.O.T.S.?

Age 13 (2008)

3.) How long did the process take? How many doctors did you have to see until you finally got an official diagnosis?

3 years to officially diagnose once symptoms started. I went through 3 different Dr. in multiple specialties such as, neuro, psych and cardiologists. Found POTS specialist through my mom's work who was doing trial studies with tilt table tests.

4.) When did you first start noticing something was wrong? First symptom or situation?

First symptom: dizziness and lightheadedness when I went from sitting/laying down to standing.

5.) Though most causes are unknown do you have any idea what might have triggered the onset of P.O.T.S.?

Puberty, considering that I am not grown out of POTS as an adult.

6.) How many trips do you take to a hospital or doctor's office per month? Per year?

Per month: 2 at the beginning because I was passing out in high school 4x a week initially. I went to hospital 3 times throughout my diagnosis due to extreme migraine. The other trip because I fell down the stairs when I passed out freshman year of high school. Last trip when I went deep-sea fishing.

7.) Do you believe you will ever fully recover from P.O.T.S. and never have any setbacks?

I currently believe that I am POTS free. I had one setback last year when I went deep-sea fishing and became extremely dehydrated from seasickness then passed out for 45 minutes. Went to hospital for fluids after that.

8.) How has this syndrome affected your work, school, relationships, and friendships? (Life in general)

I had to get an IEP in high school to be able to graduate due to multiple MD visits and leaving school early on days that I would get wiped out from passing out.

9.) What are the worst symptoms you have ever experienced caused by P.O.T.S.?

Brain fog, nausea, migraines, lightheadedness, dizziness.

10.) What has helped you recover the best? (Exercise, food diet, attitude)

Daily light exercise. Healthy eating plus salt to retain water. Drinking at least 80 Oz a day of water. Absolutely no caffeine in order to stay hydrated. Sleeping at least 9hrs at night. Staying cool in the summer and wearing compression stockings. Stockings to keep blood from pooling in legs and keeping blood in my heart/brain.

11.) What medications have you been put on to help with P.O.T.S.? Which ones worked and which ones did not?

Fludrocortisone for fluid retention. Salt tabs for water retention. Reglan for frequent nausea. Immitrex for frequent migraines. Neurotin (most used for POTS) and Zoloft for anxiety/depression from POTS. I believe they all worked very well together.

12.) Has the P.O.T.S. disease ever caused you to be depressed or feel like an outcast at any point?

Yes, I became very depressed. I never realized I was depressed until my parents told me and was put on Zoloft. I was ashamed at first however, Zoloft saved my life. Zoloft greatly reduced my panic attacks and periods of depression. I am now off all medications after 8 years and doing great. I have learned how to deal with my anxiety and no longer get depressed.

13.) To all those dealing with P.O.T.S. what would be the best advice you could give them to cope with everything that this syndrome entails?

Don't let POTS define who you are. Never stop doing what you love. Always add extra salt and water to your diet. Never lay around at home when you can be out with friends. Even when you are feeling bad, stay busy.

14.) Do you believe there needs to be more awareness brought worldwide in regards to Postural Orthostatic Tachycardia Syndrome?

In high school, I raised a lot of awareness through staff and friends. It's very important to raise awareness in schools because teens cover the largest population of POTS. There is always more room for awareness. Awareness is what will decrease diagnosis time and improve the lives of people with POTS. Finally, being diagnosed with POTS got me through the "invisible disease" quicker in order to get through high school and move onto college. I now have a college degree and am working in the field that I love because of my POTS specialist Dr. Geoffrey Heyer of Columbus, OH.

Colleen, 49 Years Old

1.) First tell me a little bit about yourself? (Name, age, hobbies, anything interesting)

My name is Colleen. I am 49 years old. I have 5 children (All boys-mostly grown) and 3 grandchildren. I work as an office manager for a pediatric dental office, I'm a volunteer EMT and I'm going to school to become a paramedic. Almost done with that, thank God! No real time for hobbies or anything like that, but to relax, I like to read trashy romance novels. Lol. Nothing that makes me think.

2.) When you were first diagnosed with P.O.T.S.?

I wasn't officially diagnosed with POTS until 2013.

3.) How long did the process take? How many doctors did you have to see until you finally got an official diagnosis?

I started looking for answers to my "issues" in early 2012, so it took a bit over a year to get diagnosed. I think it was pretty fast because two of my children have it so it was on the radar.

4.) When did you first start noticing something was wrong? First symptom or situation?

Looking back, I have had symptoms most of my life. I was always a "sickly" child and when I was 16, I started passing out and having orthostatic hypotension with tachycardia. Back then, they knew NOTHING about POTS. I started to really investigate things and look for answers 5 years ago when I started having horrible chest pain to go with everything else. Given my age, the chest pain sort of freaked me out.

5.) Though most causes are unknown do you have any idea what might have triggered the onset of P.O.T.S.?

The chest pain began right after I had a bout of strep throat. That may have triggered it, but I don't know for sure.

6.) How many trips do you take to a hospital or doctor's office per month? Per year?

My doctor visits vary depending on my symptoms. I tend to not go unless something new comes up or for a regular checkup.

7.) Do you believe you will ever fully recover from P.O.T.S. and never have any setbacks?

I do not believe I will ever fully recover at this point.

8.) How has this syndrome affected your work, school, relationships, and friendships? (Life in general)

POTS has affected every aspect of my life. I basically have no "reserve" energy for anything but the basics.

9.) What are the worst symptoms you have ever experienced caused by P.O.T.S.?

They're all awful! But the one I hate more than any is the chest pain. It's very scary. Even knowing it's POTS related, I always wonder "what if this time it isn't?

10.) What has helped you recover the best? (Exercise, food diet, attitude)

Being careful to eat small, light meals and avoiding gluten and dairy helps some. Nothing else seems to make much difference. I don't take any meds anymore. Nothing helped and I didn't want to keep putting useless poisons in my body.

11.) What medications have you been put on to help with P.O.T.S.? Which ones worked and which ones did not?

See above. Lol.

12.) Has the P.O.T.S. disease ever caused you to be depressed or feel like an outcast at any point?

Years ago, in my teens and early 20's, I went through a period of depression because I always felt so awful but nobody ever found anything wrong with me. I felt like a hypochondriac.

13.) To all those dealing with P.O.T.S. what would be the best advice you could give them to cope with everything that this syndrome entails?

My advice would be to not give up. Keep trying different things to find what works for you. This illness is no fun, but it doesn't own you. Keep your head up and be your own advocate

14.) Do you believe there needs to be more awareness brought worldwide in regards to Postural Orthostatic Tachycardia Syndrome?

I do believe that! It is so hard to deal with health professionals and people in general that have no idea what is going on. We look like we're fine. Most tests show that we're fine. But we are not fine.

Em, 23 Years Old

1.) First tell me a little bit about yourself? (Name, age, hobbies, anything interesting)

My name is Em and I'm 23 years old. I am on track for a PhD and hoping to work as an emergency doctor in a hospital someday. I have a neurological phenomenon called synesthesia and before I became ill I was a high-

*fashion model, competitive swimmer and working with
horses. I love being outdoors, reading, creating art,
writing, playing my piano and I'm also terrible at
introductions!"*

2.) When you were first diagnosed with P.O.T.S.?

I was formally diagnosed with POTS 7 April, 2016.

**3.) How long did the process take? How many doctors
did you have to see until you finally got an official
diagnosis?**

*The process took a few years. I knew I had
dysautonomia starting August of 2014, but I didn't know
where to start looking for a good doctor that would listen
to me. I was also a university student, so I wasn't able to go
to many doctor's appointments. I researched autonomic
specialists devoutly until I found one I thought I could trust.
So it only took one neurologist to diagnose me.*

**4.) When did you first start noticing something was
wrong? First symptom or situation?**

*I first noticed something was wrong my freshman
year of university. I donated plasma twice a week and they
take standing vitals. You have to be within a certain range
in order to donate. As time went on, they started turning me
away because my heart rate was too high. I didn't
understand why or that anything might be wrong. Once I
transferred schools in 2014, I started passing out several
times a day and that's when I knew something was really
wrong.*

**5.) Though most causes are unknown do you have any
idea what might have triggered the onset of P.O.T.S.?**

I do. My POTS was caused by a combination of
autoimmune disease and the Epstein-Barr virus.

6.) How many trips do you take to a hospital or doctor's office per month? Per year?

I see a neurologist 3-4 times per year. I visit my PCP at least once per month and I'm in the ER at least once per month for fluids and blood tests. I've been hospitalized twice since October of 2016 and I have various other specialists that I see. Those visits really vary, but I see them anytime from once per month to a few times per year.

7.) Do you believe you will ever fully recover from P.O.T.S. and never have any setbacks?

I hope so, but I'm honestly not holding my breath. Even if I get to the point I can lead a near-normal life, I know the possibility of regression and flares, however small, is astronomical.

8.) How has this syndrome affected your work, school, relationships, and friendships? (Life in general).

I have pretty severe POTS and two other forms of dysautonomia on top of it. It's affected my life greatly. I had to drop out of university because I'm currently too ill to attend. I have a lot of neurological symptoms, including gait disturbance, so I need a cane to walk most of the time. I had to stop modelling, camping, hiking, working with horses, sports; everything that I use to love and be very active in. My fiancé has become my primary caretaker, which I hate. I would love to be more active and go running or camping with him and I just can't right now. Friendships are a little odd because my best friend lives six hours away and has the same illnesses I do, so we have a great friendship. My closes friend geologically is an hour away. So it's convenient in the fact that I don't feel awful for not going out with friends who are always around, but it's also very, very lonely.

9.) What are the worst symptoms you have ever experienced caused by P.O.T.S.?

Well as I mentioned above, I have a lot of neurological symptoms. Gait disturbance is a huge one because I can't walk without a cane at the moment. Heart rate variability is also hard. I've had my heart rate as low as 25bpm and as high as 210bpm and my blood pressure is always very low. My fatigue has been unbelievable, which also impacts my brain fog.

10.) What has helped you recover the best? (Exercise, food diet, attitude)

I'm still looking for that magic treatment plan! I'm actively trying to pursue IVIG so I'm hoping my new neurologist will be at least willing to talk about it. So for now it's tons of salt and fluids and being as optimistic as I can, as well as knowing where my limits are and working with them. I have a service dog that has been a godsend. He's helped me so much, both physically and mentally.

11.) What medications have you been put on to help with P.O.T.S.? Which ones worked and which ones did not?

Let's see...I've tried topomax, mestinon and midodrine. None of those worked, or they worked but gave me terrible side effects. I can't take beta blockers because my blood pressure is already very low. Oddly enough, vicodin (hydrocodone + acetominophen), which I take for chronic pain, has really been amazing for my fatigue and brain fog. Other than that, we haven't found anything that's been able to help me.

12.) Has the P.O.T.S. disease ever caused you to be depressed or feel like an outcast at any point?

It definitely has! I live in a social black hole, so I haven't experienced much of feeling like an outcast in social situations, but I do feel very left out with my family's activities. My family is a very active one. We've always been into things like hiking, backpacking and camping, and my family has been helping my parents build their own house. Since I can no longer take part in any of that, I do feel very left out. Adding to that the fact I can't currently attend university or be active like I used to, depression has been a recurring companion. I've gotten to know it very well.

13.) To all those dealing with P.O.T.S. what would be the best advice you could give them to cope with everything that this syndrome entails?

Don't give up! There are always going to be doctors who don't give you the time of day. Please learn to fight for yourselves. Your health is more important than anything else. You are in no way alone. There are so many of us out there, all fighting the same battle. There are hundreds of amazing support groups spread across social media sites. I promise you that we understand what you're going through. Lastly, educate yourselves! Learn everything you can about this illness! Understanding what is happening, how and what you can do to help yourselves is going to make all the difference.

14.) Do you believe there needs to be more awareness brought worldwide in regards to Postural Orthostatic Tachycardia Syndrome?

Absolutely! The average wait time for diagnosis is seven years. That's insane! More awareness means more medical education. There are currently so little specialists available. Some patients have to travel outside of their own country to see a doctor or get treatment and that's just unacceptable. It's expensive to have an illness that's so little known and I can't even imagine how many people are out there who are either misdiagnosed and getting the wrong treatment or have no idea what's happening to them. More education and more awareness means more education and more chance that someone, somewhere will find a cure.

Jenny, 18 Years Old

1.) First tell me a little bit about yourself? (Name, age, hobbies, anything interesting)

My name is Julianna but I go by Jenny. I'm 18; I'll be turning 19 in a few months. I'm currently in school to be an actress, but it's really hard, not just in general but on my body. Acting takes a lot of physical work.

2.) When you were first diagnosed with P.O.T.S.?

I was diagnosed when I was 16. It was the beginning of December. I still remember that.

3.) How long did the process take? How many doctors did you have to see until you finally got an official diagnosis?

I saw a cardiologist once, when I first started getting symptoms, when I was 11. But I only had one symptom back then, and we all thought it was a heart problem, not a vascular one. After being unable to diagnose me, I decided to ignore it until five years later, when I finally went back in and was diagnosed.

4.) When did you first start noticing something was wrong? First symptom or situation?

I started getting symptoms - tachycardia episodes, to begin with - when I was 10 or 11. I saw a cardiologist - the same one that would diagnose me, 5 years later - but without any structural abnormalities in my heart, she had nothing to go on. I had yet to get dizzy spells, so my only symptom was the tachycardia. She gave me a device to record an episode when it happened, but then I went three months free and returned it. I promptly began to have episodes, but being a scared, lonely preteen in the midst of family drama, school drama, friend drama, and just about every other kind of drama, I decided to ignore it so as not to bother anyone around me. I had severe self-esteem issues back then, and this story definitely shows it. It wasn't until after I had a nervous breakdown and started having fainting spells and severe dizziness that I finally admitted to my parents the attacks had never gone away. We went back to the doctor, and with all my new symptoms, she took about ten minutes to diagnose me. My main issue was that my symptoms came in backwards - I got the worst one first, then the slightly easier ones later. It confused everyone.

5.) Though most causes are unknown do you have any idea what might have triggered the onset of P.O.T.S.?

As far as we can tell, it had to do with the hormone fluctuation that came at the beginning of puberty. I was also diagnosed with Alopecia Areata and scoliosis when I was 11, so POTS wasn't the only thing that started around that time.

6.) How many trips do you take to a hospital or doctor's office per month? Per year?

I try not to visit the doctor except for check-ups or emergencies. Still, despite not really having a "per month" number, my per year number is somewhere in the high teens. Only about three of those are to my cardiologist, though. In addition to POTS, I have eczema (diagnosed as a baby), severe allergies (diagnosed as a toddler), scoliosis (noticed at 11, officially diagnosed at 16), Alopecia (diagnosed at 11), depression and anxiety (diagnosed at 15), ADHD (diagnosed as a child), a ganglion cyst in my knee that I am getting surgically removed in about a month (result of skiing accident at 11, diagnosed at 18, just about a month ago), a history of ovarian cysts, the first of which had to be surgically removed (diagnosed at 15), severe menstrual cramping as a result of the cyst surgery (diagnosed at 15), and I'm prone to accidents and get sick. All of that together adds up a lot.

7.) Do you believe you will ever fully recover from P.O.T.S. and never have any setbacks?

Do I hope I will? Absolutely. I hope that I fully recover in some miracle, or a cure is found, or a medication works for me wonderfully and I stop having symptoms. But it's not realistic. So, no, I don't believe that. I can't. Getting my hopes up too much will only disappoint me when it doesn't happen. I'm surviving, right now. If someone tells me there's a cure, and then it never comes, I don't know if I'll survive that.

8.) How has this syndrome affected your work, school, relationships, and friendships? (Life in general)

I dropped out of school less than three months after getting diagnosed. I got my GED a year later. Right now, I'm in trade school, so that I can graduate in a little more than a year, rather than go to a four-year school that I know I wouldn't survive. I do my best, but it's hard, when people don't understand what it's like. One of my teachers always praises this graduate who had some sort of severe bowel problem, and another who had kidney disease, both of whom "never complained". I don't know what happened to bowel boy, but kidney boy just fucking died. I mean, who praises someone who just died for not complaining about the excruciating pain he was in while in school? I always want to tell the teacher to fuck off. If he truly understood what it was like to be chronically ill, he'd never say anything like that. But I can't say anything. I just have to listen to him praise a dead kid.

9.) What are the worst symptoms you have ever experienced caused by P.O.T.S.?

Definitely the tachycardia. I can survive dizziness, the fainting gets better once I lie down for a few minutes, but the tachycardia comes unexpectedly, and painfully. I hate it so much.

10.) What has helped you recover the best? (Exercise, food diet, attitude)

I'd say learning to get enough sleep helped the most. I was severely sleep deprived for years, then after dropping out, I was suddenly sleeping as much as I could, and I felt amazing. Now, I try to get a good 10 hours a

*night if possible, with more on the weekends. Sometimes I
sleep up to 15 hours. It's awesome.*

**11.) What medications have you been put on to help
with P.O.T.S.? Which ones worked and which ones did
not?**

*I mostly take supplements that were recommended
by my doctors. So iron, vitamin B, and vitamin B. The B I
take every morning, and it does help with energy. The D
and iron are new enough that if they are going to have an
effect, I haven't felt it yet.*

**12.) Has the P.O.T.S. disease ever caused you to be
depressed or feel like an outcast at any point?**

*All the time. I ended up in a mental hospital for four
months due to severe depression. So, yeah. All the time.*

**13.) To all those dealing with P.O.T.S. what would be
the best advice you could give them to cope with
everything that this syndrome entails?**

*What advice can I give? Don't give up, it might get
better? That's bullshit. Drink more water? True, but
annoying to always hear. Soy sauce is your life now?
Actually, that one may be helpful. Soy sauce is life. And
God. "And Jesus. And the Dalai Llama. Combined. I
recommend all Potsies learn to worship soy sauce.*

**14.) Do you believe there needs to be more awareness
brought worldwide in regards to Postural Orthostatic
Tachycardia Syndrome?**

*I believe there are a lot of things that need more
awareness, and POTS is definitely one of them. I'm*

actually really fucking lucky. I have great parents, I'm well off, and I can go to school and get a job and have a life. There are so many of us that can't. And then we're called lazy. I never want to strangle someone quite as much as when they call one of us "lazy".

Chris, 25 Years Old

1.) First tell me a little bit about yourself? (Name, age, hobbies, anything interesting)

My actual name is Chris (The DMX DJ is my artist name), I am 25 years old and live in a small market town called Stamford in Lincolnshire (UK). My background before my diagnosis is that I was a professional lighting technician for my local nightclub ensuring an awesome atmosphere during every song played, I worked alongside some of the biggest and best music artists in the UK music industry, from ultrabeat, the wideboys, the clubland franchise, Radio1 and Ibiza uncovered, i also worked on my local funfairs from time to time just because it was an awesome time with awesome people.

2.) When you were first diagnosed with P.O.T.S.?

"I first came down with a viral infection on the 19th of May 2013 that is believed to have kick-started the dysautonomia but was officially diagnosed on the 23rd December 2014.

3.) How long did the process take? How many doctors did you have to see until you finally got an official diagnosis?

It was an awfully long process of being passed back and forth through different doctors trying to figure out what was wrong, I had 5 different GP's and 2 specialists all taking guesses and trying to work it out but interestingly it was a phone call from an uncle who is a doctor himself that set me on the right path, he rang me and said, "do you have, 'list of symptoms", to which I was surprised he listed practically all of my symptoms and told me he thinks it is P.O.T.S, when I went back to my own doctor I told him about this and ordered a Tilt table test which confirmed my diagnosis.

4.) When did you first start noticing something was wrong? First symptom or situation?

The first sign something was wrong was when i got up to go to work on that morning of the 19th May 2013 when I noticed my heart was beating a lot faster than it should have been, i generally ignored it and went to work as normal, as the morning went on i was slowly feeling breathless and dizzy, I got through it until i came back in from a cigarette break and suddenly lost all control of myself, i was pale, had no strength and collapsed at work.

5.) Though most causes are unknown do you have any idea what might have triggered the onset of P.O.T.S.?

Yes, I believe that in my case it was a mixture of energy drink consumption and cleaning chemicals at work, the energy drinks because of the increased adrenal secretion over a long period of time, and the cleaning products because they could have easily started attacking my immune system.

6.) How many trips do you take to a hospital or doctor's office per month? Per year?

Honestly I don't anymore, because they still pass me from pillar to post and there is no cure, I have taken it upon myself to do things my own way, I am always researching ways of improving my condition and look into the research that has been going on into POTS Dysautonomia.

7.) Do you believe you will ever fully recover from P.O.T.S. and never have any setbacks?

I don't believe I will recover fully, everything you try and do (with drugs) causes other symptoms to arise, if you exercise, although it is supposed to help it doesn't because any exertion makes everything a lot worse. With our condition, everything seems to be a catch 22 situation.

8.) How has this syndrome affected your work, school, relationships, and friendships? (Life in general)

I cannot work, I cannot even tolerate being stood up for 10 minutes, let alone walk long distances, the most i can walk without a rest is about 300 meters. I still talk to people online but generally I don't go out much at all and will not allow people to see me at my worst. I have indeed lost friendships because of my condition but if they are too narrow minded to see that you can be sick on the inside and look ok on the outside then as far as I see it's really not my problem. I even got accused of attention seeking when trying to explain what this condition is and what it does to you. I have no time for those sorts of people but all the time in the world for someone who wants to know and open their minds. I lost my girlfriend because of my own train of thought. I broke up with her because I didn't feel it was fair on her to be constantly worried and not be able to go out on days out and dates, even intimacy and 'doing the deed' was a no go most of the time because of the effects on my health.

9.) What are the worst symptoms you have ever experienced caused by P.O.T.S.?

The worst things that have happened to me was the sensation of having a stroke and a heart attack simultaneously, yet when it came to the ECG/EKG it came back with no sign of infarction, they still rushed me in as my heart-rate although lying flat kept a fluctuation between 75bpm and 230bpm, my oxygen levels were rising, falling and the shots of pain shooting through my body that were overpowering. It was a very strange sensation because I felt like I was already dead, but then rationally I thought I can feel.... I'm not dead... what in the world is going on? (It was a physical feeling, not anxiety) I do not get anxious with these attacks because I have prepared myself that one day it could kill me (there have been cases of sudden cardiac death and respiratory arrest in dysautonomia).

10.) What has helped you recover the best? (Exercise, food diet, attitude)

The things that have helped me the most is: getting rid of the people in my life that cause me problems, whether it be because they are too ignorant to see the truth that is dysautonomia, they are general troublemakers and people who overall have a negative effect on me which has kept me in a more positive mindset. Allowing my body to dictate to me what i can and can't do, I do not encourage me to push the barriers of my capabilities.

11.) What medications have you been put on to help with P.O.T.S.? Which ones worked and which ones did not?

I do not take medication, every medicine I have been on had a negative effect, from causing added symptoms to masking my capabilities (I would often do more than my body could handle while on medication, when the medicine wore off, I'd have a really bad time with it). So, without medication I can gauge my capabilities a lot more accurately.

12.) Has the P.O.T.S. disease ever caused you to be depressed or feel like an outcast at any point?

Absolutely, I have often thought about taking my own life because having dysautonomia is no way to live a life, but being on Facebook and so other groups involved with the condition and knowing that there are so many people going through it opens my eyes when I think this way because we are all battling it together, we share stories, advice, and are genuinely the best people I know, every person with dysautonomia is open minded and has a wider view of the world in general because of the 'cards they were dealt' in life. if I took my own life, we wouldn't be talking now and I wouldn't be giving my story to you, any publicity which gets dysautonomia seen and read about is good, the more people that know, the better it can be researched and the more people will want to research it and find a cure.

13.) To all those dealing with P.O.T.S. what would be the best advice you could give them to cope with everything that this syndrome entails?

I would say join the groups, get advice from the people living with it, no doctor will understand our condition like we do unless they live with it themselves. It is important to keep your loved ones close, do not be afraid to ask anything, be as open and honest as you can. Even ask the smallest questions getting on your nerves, if it's to do with the digestive system, intimate things that we are often embarrassed about, ask them, honestly no one will judge. We are all in the same boat and understand these things. POTS UK and Dysautonomia International are great sources of information and do amazing work to help find a cure; it's also worth a look at UCLA and the mayo clinic for the latest in research.

14.) Do you believe there needs to be more awareness brought worldwide in regards to Postural Orthostatic Tachycardia Syndrome?

Absolutely, dysautonomias in general need a lot more awareness, I have even done my bit, I created a music album which is now on iTunes and all of the major online music stores called POTS Awareness, all of the proceeds of that album go to POTS UK to raise awareness and help find a cure, i will continue to do as much as I can to help people like us, even being there as someone who listens helps people in our situation, many feel alone, opening up to someone helps which is why I try to be as active as i can, I am no psychiatrist but just being there for someone is the best feeling in the world.

Bethany, 23 Years Old

1.) **First tell me a little bit about yourself? (Name, age, hobbies, anything interesting)**

I'm Bethany, I'm 23. My hobbies are singing and anything musical, reading and creative writing. I studied health care at college till I got ill but was planning to be a psychologist.

2.) When you were first diagnosed with P.O.T.S.?

I was diagnosed in August of 2016.

3.) How long did the process take? How many doctors did you have to see until you finally got an official diagnosis?

It's taken almost my whole life; I've had symptoms of POTS since a very young age and have been to 11 doctors including a psychiatrist after being labelled an attention seeker.

4.) When did you first start noticing something was wrong? First symptom or situation?

When it became clear something was very wrong besides ME/Fibromyalgia is when I began having severe tremors and fainted for the first time shortly after a car accident in 2014.

5.) Though most causes are unknown do you have any idea what might have triggered the onset of P.O.T.S.?

I was diagnosed with Ehlers-Danlos Syndrome type 3 at the same time as the POTS and was told that is the cause.

6.) How many trips do you take to a hospital or doctor's office per month? Per year?

I see my cardiologist every 2 months and occasionally go to ER because I faint daily and often get hurt.

7.) Do you believe you will ever fully recover from P.O.T.S. and never have any setbacks?

*My cardiologist said that because I began
symptoms in my twenties that I will not grow out of it and
will most likely decline with age.*

**8.) How has this syndrome affected your work, school,
relationships, and friendships? (Life in general)**

*I had to give up what little work my fatigue allowed
once I started fainting. My friends all left me very quickly
and my social life has ended very abruptly. And as for
relationships like dating, I've not yet found a boyfriend who
can tolerate my symptoms. And it's also put a strain on my
family life as certain family believed I was attention
seeking and my parents struggle to cope with me being as
ill as I am.*

**9.) What are the worst symptoms you have ever
experienced caused by P.O.T.S.?**

*I think the daily fainting is one of the worst but I
recently had around 40 anoxic seizures after a faint one
after the other and I thought I was going to die; I was
exhausted, in pain and scared. I think that is the worst time
I've ever had.*

**10.) What has helped you recover the best? (Exercise,
food diet, attitude)**

*I'm determined to remain positive despite my
symptoms and struggles and I find light exercise at times
helps, not always but I love doing yoga. Avoiding carbs like
potato, rice and pasta has helped symptoms hugely too.*

**11.) What medications have you been put on to help
with P.O.T.S.? Which ones worked and which ones did
not?**

I have so far taken Ivabradine and Porpranalol both of which have been stopped because of intolerable side effects such as increased palpitations and chest tightness. So at this point nothing has helped.

12.) Has the P.O.T.S. disease ever caused you to be depressed or feel like an outcast at any point?

*Yes. I've always suffered with depression and self-harming but it's got a lot **lot** worse in the last 18 months. None of my friends have stood by me and I feel like an outcast and completely alone.*

13.) To all those dealing with P.O.T.S. what would be the best advice you could give them to cope with everything that this syndrome entails?

Take it one day at a time. Never push your limits and stick to the people who love you.

14.) Do you believe there needs to be more awareness brought worldwide in regards to Postural Orthostatic Tachycardia Syndrome?

Very much so! I've dealt with loads of doctors/paramedics/nurses who give me a blank stare when I say POTS and I have to explain it and it is not rare. The ignorance around POTS needs to end.

Christine, 43 Years Old

1.) First tell me a little bit about yourself? (Name, age, hobbies, anything interesting)

My name is Christine, I am 43 years old. I was married young and had 3 children in the first 5 years, so we now have 3 adult children, one son-in-law and two adorable granddaughters. I live in a quaint small city in Manitoba Canada, in a cute old 2 story house, with two of our kids and 2 dogs. I have a Para Educator Certificate and have worked with special needs children of all ages. I specialized in speech therapy. I love to read, draw, write and play piano!

2.) When you were first diagnosed with P.O.T.S.?

I was diagnosed with POTS in 2012 by a cardiologist who did the poor man's tilt. She did an official Tilt Table Test in 2015 as one was available then, and confirmed classic POTS without a shadow of a doubt!

3.) How long did the process take? How many doctors did you have to see until you finally got an official diagnosis?

I got very sick (dizzy, vertigo, shaking, nauseas, short of breath- my face and lips were blueish) quite suddenly and had to be rushed to the ER from the school I was working at. I saw 2 or 3 doctors that day that diagnosed low iron, high blood pressure and dehydration. I left the hospital after IV fluids with a prescription for iron, and Atenolol. My family doctor then tested me for pheochromocytoma (tumors on the adrenal glands) as I had no previous history of high blood pressure. When that was negative, I had a MRI, CT scan, and many blood tests for Lupus, and thyroid issues among other things. He referred me to a neurologist, who incorrectly diagnosed an inner ear problem, and an internal medical specialist who suspected POTS among other options, and sent me to the Cardiologist. The cardiologist then diagnosed POTS almost exactly one year after I first got so sick!

4.) When did you first start noticing something was wrong? First symptom or situation?

I first noticed symptoms of tachycardia and PVC's in grade 5 when standing to sing the national anthem in school! I would also get very short of breath doing any running, and I would feel my heart race. The doctors at that time diagnosed me with a heart murmur caused by a prolapsed valve. They felt it caused my PVC's and mild tachycardia. They told me it would "not affect my life." I just lived with the symptoms, but fatigue and brain fog plagued my teen years. I was not at all athletic!!! I lived relatively normally though until about 2006 when the fatigue was so bad I quit my job, and started having episodes of shaking and shortness of breath. I also was having swollen ankles, and would have to lie down with my feet up on pillows in the evenings. My doctor wondered if my kidneys were maybe damaged from a bad infection I had a few years before. I was also told to lose weight. After 2 years off I went back to work and plugged through the worsening fatigue, lay down all evening every evening, and rested all weekend, until my body completely broke down that day at school in November of 2011. I cannot work at all now- doctors' orders!

5.) Though most causes are unknown do you have any idea what might have triggered the onset of P.O.T.S.?

I feel that POTS was in my DNA, and I developed the mild symptoms at the age of 11 when I hit puberty- but the sudden onsets of the extreme symptoms were caused by stress. I had an alcoholic supervisor at the time, and a student who I had to stop from attempting suicide in the washroom while in my care. The school was overcrowded and not properly managed. I had 3 teenagers at home and a troubled marriage at the time.

6.) How many trips do you take to a hospital or doctor's office per month? Per year?

I see my family doctor every 3 or 4 months, and my Cardiologist 2 times a year.

7.) Do you believe you will ever fully recover from P.O.T.S. and never have any setbacks?

I believe I will always have at least a mild form of POTS, but I hope the symptoms will become as mild as they were in my 20's! If I stay on my beta blocker, (I am now on Propanol instead of Atenolol) and stay hydrated, getting a lot of rest) I hope to resume working part time. My cardiologist said she can never see me going back to work full time.

8.) How has this syndrome affected your work, school, relationships, and friendships? (Life in general)

I am basically housebound. I can manage my symptoms in my own home, where I can rest whenever I need to, sit or lay down suddenly if I need to and avoid fainting. I am partially functioning as a "housewife" at home, lying down periodically throughout the day, sitting on stools in the kitchen, really limiting anything strenuous like vacuuming or carrying laundry. I cannot do yard work. I shop online. I have great relationships with my family now, and I feel like I am always there for them. They can talk to me whenever they need to and they can rely on me for advice, etc. I have my parents over a couple of times a year and I can go to their house a few times a year. But my friendships have suffered. I don't have energy to entertain. The odd time I have tried to get together with friends I have had to leave when I feel like passing out. I don't have energy to have friends come visit. I have a few friends who understand this and we keep close through Facebook, texts and Emails! I appreciate that so much!!! One friend snail mail's me cute cards and letters and have an Aunt who phones me once a month or so. These ladies mean so much to me! They understand I cannot go visit them or don't have the energy to have company, yet they keep up with me!! I cannot drive due to the vertigo.

9.) What are the worst symptoms you have ever experienced caused by P.O.T.S.?

The worst symptom is the presyncope. The feeling that I will pass out or collapse if I don't immediately lay down. It makes me afraid to leave the house.

10.) What has helped you recover the best? (Exercise, food diet, attitude)

Pacing myself and realizing my body's limitations has helped me the most. Realizing that if I push myself too much and overdo it too much it can take WEEKS to recover- it pushes me backwards! My cardiologist always reminds me to lay down and rest BEFORE I feel like I will keel over. I do a chore, then rest, prepare some food, then rest, sit up and talk with a family member, then rest...... it also helps me to avoid spicy and acidic foods. I don't know why, (and neither do my doctors,) but digesting something like Salsa for example causes much worse symptoms in me! It is also hard for me to digest raw vegetables. So if I were to eat a taco salad for example, I would have exaggerated symptoms of dizziness, shortness of breath, shaking and presyncope while it digests. Eating bland, easy to digest foods makes a positive difference for me!! It also helps to focus on what I CAN do instead of dwelling on what I CAN't do!!

11.) What medications have you been put on to help with P.O.T.S.? Which ones worked and which ones did not?

Atenolol lowered my blood pressure too much after a year of it working perfectly for me. I then tried Metoprolol and Bisoprolol which lowered my heart rate too much (40's)! I tried Diltiazem which raised my heart rate to 150 resting!! And raised my blood pressure, also giving me stroke like symptoms!!! (I called 911 because I thought I was having a stroke after my second dose). I finally tried a low dose (15 mg 3x a day) of Propanolol, and it keeps my heart rate under 120, keeps my blood pressure normal, and helps me to overall to feel a bit better. I feel calmer and less headaches and dizziness.

12.) Has the P.O.T.S. disease ever caused you to be depressed or feel like an outcast at any point?

I have felt left out whenever my husband and kids go somewhere I can't. They usually plan things I can do too- in a climate controlled place that I can sit down.....but once in a while I feel deeply left out. I have struggled with depression my whole life.....I cope without medication, my faith in God, believing he has a purpose and a plan for me helps A LOT!!!!

13.) To all those dealing with P.O.T.S. what would be the best advice you could give them to cope with everything that this syndrome entails?

My advice would be: Realize that your body is different now! Your life is different now! Accept your new normal! Grieve the loss of your previous life, but realize you have a NEW purpose! (I have taken up writing, as well as more time for hobbies.

14.) Do you believe there needs to be more awareness brought worldwide in regards to Postural Orthostatic Tachycardia Syndrome?

Yes more health care professionals need to be taught about POTS!!! My family doctor had never heard of it! Most ER doctors have never heard of it! I have to explain what it is to all the nurses- My daughter is just graduating from nursing as an LPN and Dysautonomia was not even covered!! At the very least it should be described in textbooks! I think the "public" is learning more and more about POTS through social media and that is great!!! I also have talked to many people who know of someone in their circle who has POTS. So even if it's just, "Oh the lady that used to work at the florist's has POTS." So more and more people all the time are at least familiar with the name! Or "My coworker's sister in law has POTS." There have also been a few Stories on the 6 o'clock news about people with POTS. So more and more people all the time are at least familiar with the name!

Lisa, 31 Years Old

1.) First tell me a little bit about yourself? (Name, age, hobbies, anything interesting)

Lisa Swanson, 31 yrs. old, I enjoy doing stuff with my children and working on our house.

2.) When you were first diagnosed with P.O.T.S.?

I was diagnosed with POTS at the age of 30. I did not do a tilt table test, but they monitored my pulse after I told her when I switched positions I would feel like passing out.

3.) How long did the process take? How many doctors did you have to see until you finally got an official diagnosis?

This was the first doctor I had ever spoken to about this and right away when I mentioned my symptoms she monitored my pulse and BP.

4.) When did you first start noticing something was wrong? First symptom or situation?

I started noticing symptoms as a young child, around the age 6 or so. The first thing I remember is when I got out of bed to fast I would black out so I had to take my time. I also knew I was sensitive to heat and light. When I was young and my mom would blow dry my hair I would have to lay down often because my heart would race and I would start to black out and get dizzy.

5.) Though most causes are unknown do you have any idea what might have triggered the onset of P.O.T.S.?

This was something I believe I was born with. I also suffer from Uticaria, had issues with this right along with POTS. My neurologist did blood work and urine test and said I have mild Mastocytosis.

6.) How many trips do you take to a hospital or doctor's office per month? Per year?

I go to the doctor about 4 times a year. I have my annual apt and then I see a neurologist twice a year.

7.) Do you believe you will ever fully recover from P.O.T.S. and never have any setbacks?

No, I will have this problem till I die. I feel it has gotten worse since I've gotten older. I am more sensitive to heat, lights and have to take my time walking up stairs etc.

8.) How has this syndrome affected your work, school, relationships, and friendships? (Life in general)

I can't go outside and play with my kids when it's super-hot because I get sick. I have become more of a homebody because I never know when I will get nauseous and have to lay down from food. Sometimes I feel cheated since I worry more than the average person. For example, I was in a wedding a few years back and had extra anxiety because I kept thinking if it's too bright or hot I am going to just pass out. Also how do you explain when your husband asks you to hold something on the wall that you can't hold your hands up longer than 10 seconds? Doing hairstyles is also very hard. For instance, watching COPS on TV and they have to put their hands in the air, the first thing I think of is well if they have POTS they probably can't hold their arms up for longer than a minute.

9.) What are the worst symptoms you have ever experienced caused by P.O.T.S.?

Increased heart rate. When I get a stomach ache it spikes so high, especially the stomach flu. I have to craw to the toilet. I fear getting sick when I'm older. Before I was diagnosed with POTS I had my gallbladder taken out. After my surgery when I sat up to put my shirt on my pulse would sky rocket and of course the nurse wasn't in the room at the time. It took me an hour with my husband's help to put it on. I had to be wheel chaired out and lay flat in the vehicle till I got home. I know if the nurse saw my pulse and BP I wouldn't have been released home. It took almost a week for my pulse and blood pressure to go down. At that time I didn't know what was happening because I hadn't been diagnosed. I had to sleep sitting up because of the spasms and gas pain. Well, then when I would stand up or try and lay down my heart would race so high and my BP went up. I actually called my surgeon and he said I had "anxiety" and I was fine. I kept thinking what is wrong with me?!!!! I know it's not anxiety but what else could it be? My husband had to take extra time off from work because I couldn't function and take care of my kids. After about 4 days I started finally feeling like myself. Now I know next time I ever need surgery or anesthesia I will tell them about POTS and hopefully they will know about this.

10.) What has helped you recover the best? (Exercise, food diet, attitude)

Laying down and trying to remind myself that it could be worse. I have to take it easy with exercise and overheating myself.

11.) What medications have you been put on to help with P.O.T.S.? Which ones worked and which ones did not?

None. Only medication I take is Zyrtec to help with my Uticaria.

12.) Has the P.O.T.S. disease ever caused you to be depressed or feel like an outcast at any point?

Gives me anxiety and in turn that can be depressing. I always have to see how hot it will be, I have to be inside sometimes when everyone is out having fun. When I try to explain it I feel like people think I am complaining and exaggerating.

13.) To all those dealing with P.O.T.S. what would be the best advice you could give them to cope with everything that this syndrome entails?

Everyone's experiences may be different. Take it day by day.

14.) Do you believe there needs to be more awareness brought worldwide in regards to Postural Orthostatic Tachycardia Syndrome?

Yes definitely!!! I was so stoked to see if featured on the Doctors, but it was such a short lived clip. Also, when I enter my symptoms into Web Md, POTS doesn't pop up. We need more awareness. I had no idea what I had my whole life, just that it's different and normal for me. And having social media is amazing because I don't feel alone!!!!!

Emily, 20 Years Old

1.) First tell me a little bit about yourself? (Name, age, hobbies, anything interesting)

Emily just turned 20! I'm from Syracuse, NY (Go Orange!!) and the oldest of 4 kids. I'm Biochemistry major at Skidmore College and hope to go to medical school to become a Pediatrician. I'm an EMT and I volunteer with our agency on campus. I'm also a tour guide, Peer Health Educator, President of SkidEats club (food sustainability and food appreciation), and I do research in the Chemistry department in our analytical lab. We are working on building cost-effective urine based malaria diagnostic!! I also love baking cupcakes and running.

2.) When you were first diagnosed with P.O.T.S.?

My Pediatrician brought up the idea when I was about 14 but all my "tests" were "negative" (I'm not quite sure about this looking back but nothing I can do about it now). I was officially diagnosed with POTS from a tilt table test in January of 2016 (so pretty much one year ago) with new doctors in Saratoga Springs, NY.

3.) How long did the process take? How many doctors did you have to see until you finally got an official diagnosis?

I saw a cardiologist at home when I was 14 and their testing came back negative-- they never did a TTT though. I have seen many doctors including three cardiologists, one neurologist, my pediatrician when I was younger, and now my primary care doctor after I switched. I also saw a concussion specialist from having so many concussions from fainting because of POTs. The whole process took about 7 or 8 years I would say.

4.) When did you first start noticing something was wrong? First symptom or situation?

I started fainting when I was about 12 or 13. It definitely could have been long before that and I just thought the symptoms were from other illnesses.

5.) Though most causes are unknown do you have any

idea what might have triggered the onset of P.O.T.S.?

I had a mono like illness (some mono tests were positive some negative. Different doctors say different things) when I was 10 and it kept me out of school for 5 months and part of the summer. Ever since then I have been unhealthy (always getting sick, always tired, headache every single day) and POTs progressed. Not sure if this has anything to do with it or just a coincidence.

6.) How many trips do you take to a hospital or doctor's office per month? Per year?

When I'm doing "well" I have gone a month without the hospital or doctor, but for example this past September and October while at college I ended up in the hospital 3 times and saw my various doctors probably 6-8 times in about 30 days (not including being on the phone with them almost every day). In the past year since I have been diagnosed I have been to the hospital 4 times, Urgent care 2 times, and various doctors' offices probably between 30 and 40 times I've honestly lost count. It takes so much time away from my studying and college work. I have to balance having doctors in different cities depending on if I'm at school or home.

7.) Do you believe you will ever fully recover from P.O.T.S. and never have any setbacks?

I am hopeful that I will be able to get POTS under control enough to live with it at a functional level but I don't think I'll ever fully recover and have no setbacks.

8.) How has this syndrome affected your work, school, relationships, and friendships? (Life in general)

POTS has completely affected all aspects of my life. Last semester I had to drop out of classes and almost had to take a medical leave and go home. This semester I am already struggling with a reduced course load and it is only the second week in. Going from Valedictorian of my high school to not being able to keep up with college school work (I have a headache or migraine almost every day, can't concentrate, and my memory is now terrible) is devastating and emotionally really challenging. My friends try to understand and some of them are the reason I am here today. They have supported me through it all, taken me to the hospital and doctors' offices (since I'm away from my parents at school), and encouraged me with everything. They make me rest when I need to and support me in any way they can. Some friends, however, don't understand at all and make fun of me when I can't participate in certain social activities or go out partying with them. They don't understand why I'm always in the library struggling to get all my work done when they've been done for hours. It's really frustrating especially coming to college and being diagnosed with POTS my freshman year. I had a flare up less than 2 months into my freshman year and then again fall of this year (my sophomore year). I miss out on a lot of things and am not able to experience what others are able to take advantage of. I pretty much have to struggle every day to just stay 'healthy" and keep moving forward which is something others just take for granted.

9.) What are the worst symptoms you have ever experienced caused by P.O.T.S.?

Fainting and waking up by myself having no idea where I am, how I got there, or how long I have been unconscious for. Also having a headache or migraine every single day of my life since I was about 14.

10.) What has helped you recover the best? (Exercise, food diet, attitude)

Fludrocortisone by far. Drinking 4 Liters of water per day and taking 8-10g of salt tablets. Trying to run every morning (when I am able to) has helped to get my blood flowing and help me faint less.

11.) What medications have you been put on to help with P.O.T.S.? Which ones worked and which ones did not?

I've been put on so many I don't even remember them all. I also have migraines so I have tried a lot (unsuccessfully). Most recently I have been on Midodrine, Bisoprolol, and Fludrocortisone. Bisoprolol was awful, Midodrine was so-so, and Fludrocortisone has improved my symptoms significantly.

12.) Has the P.O.T.S. disease ever caused you to be depressed or feel like an outcast at any point?

Yes it prevents me from doing a lot of social things and people often don't understand. Since it is "invisible" people don't even think I'm sick sometimes. I spent most of this past semester really depressed and upset almost every day. Some days I really am okay and other days I just feel like I can't go on.

13.) To all those dealing with P.O.T.S. what would be the best advice you could give them to cope with everything that this syndrome entails?

Find a good support system it is everything. Don't give up even when it feels like everything is falling apart and you will never recover. It will have its ups and downs but it means you are living and moving forward one day at a time.

14.) Do you believe there needs to be more awareness brought worldwide in regards to Postural Orthostatic Tachycardia Syndrome?

YES!! More awareness, support, and RESEARCH!!!

Taylor, 18 Years Old

1.) First tell me a little bit about yourself? (Name, age, hobbies, anything interesting)

My name is Taylor. I am 18 years old. Some hobbies of mine are singing, long distance running and acting.

2.) When you were first diagnosed with P.O.T.S.?

I was first diagnosed with POTS in May I want to say of 2016. It took a year to get diagnosed.

3.) How long did the process take? How many doctors did you have to see until you finally got an official diagnosis?

It did take a year to learn that I had POTS. I saw 5 doctors that year and was about to look for more. 2 out of those 5 doctors were not so bad.

4.) When did you first start noticing something was wrong? First symptom or situation?

I started to notice something was wrong after I couldn't do normal actions or focus clearly. It took me out of school and it hit me a lot harder than my anorexia recovery did. I would feel like passing out and I couldn't stand up straight. I would feel tired constantly and very weak. I knew that this wasn't normal. Especially when I couldn't do the things I loved.

5.) Though most causes are unknown do you have any idea what might have triggered the onset of P.O.T.S.?

Definitely my anorexia that was an ongoing issue and got worse due to my POTS. It was hard to keep up with food always feeling sick. I posted a story on my Facebook that is the first post. It explains a lot of my own story. The research I did add up to a possible cure. Howeve,r it wouldn't apply to everyone. I am getting better because of what I researched. I do want to post what helped me out sometime soon. The sad thing that did pop up was that a lot of these people now rely on a bunch of things to keep them going. Whether it is meds or tubes. After that long time frame the body could take many years to heal even if they have an overall cure.

6.) How many trips do you take to a hospital or doctor's office per month? Per year?

I go around once to twice a month. It was never more than that unfortunately I was so sick yet had to wait forever for doctors to see me. This in turn builds up the time frame. Labs are the last thing to show something. But doctors rely on it so heavily. Per year I can't even imagine. I had a lot of hospital stays for when I couldn't take care of myself. Even the staff didn't believe I was sick.

7.) Do you believe you will ever fully recover from P.O.T.S. and never have any setbacks?

Nothing is set in stone but this is a real illness. Trust me it takes it's time. I am improving but there is no way to tell until I am actually healthy again. I do have some hope that I can defeat this. If I were not able to... well I am glad I fought despite the odds.

8.) How has this syndrome affected your work, school, relationships, and friendships? (Life in general)

HA! All of my relationships and everything about my life changed. Some for the better because they never supported me. But It definitely made things arduous. I had more problems with trying to keep friendships alive. My schooling was so hard on me. People in places of authority and my ex friends didn't believe I was sick enough. My family for a while was unsure. Until it got worse. Isolation tends to be a trend we all have as people growing up with POTS. It is the second worst to the illness itself. You get misunderstood a lot. Most times isolation is there because many don't even know the illness or understand it. Most likely no one will know you have it unless you tell them. It is called an invisible illness for a reason. It stopped me in

119

my tracks and the possibilities to pay for school. This is why I can't afford college now. It has made everything automatically more demanding. Even the things I love to do.

9.) What are the worst symptoms you have ever experienced caused by P.O.T.S.?

When it made me weak enough to not be able to feed myself. My vision was in and out and my energy was beyond destroyed. I was in a wheel chair for some time too. There is no easy way with pots. People talking like you can easily get out without even having the illness don't even know what they're asking the person to feel and do. It made my anorexia worse. Another myth is that this illness doesn't kill you. But wouldn't it? Considering how much it disables you? It was the domino that made all the other dominos fall. That was this illness. I only got sicker at the time. It made me sick enough so that I couldn't look at screens. I would lie down all day in pain. It's sad that most of us potsie's have to pick ourselves up from such a demanding place. That you shouldn't be alone for. The symptoms I had are also on my story. It was this feeling of waves(like electricity) running from my neck to my legs throughout my entire body. I would get flares at random times. Still do and I can't do much on those days. When that wave hits you, you are weak and shaky. Circulation is bad and your fingers/legs/ feet are purple. Your stomach is all wacky. You can't focus as much as you want to. You forget things and have to remind yourself constantly. Or you completely forget. The stress that comes with having this illness is a package deal.

10.) What has helped you recover the best? (Exercise, food diet, attitude)

Well it wasn't one single doctor I can tell you that. And having the best attitude in the world won't cure this. But it will help you to find your own answers. It helped me find mine at my sickest. All on my story as well. Exercise can only help so much. I hate that they pressure that the most. Like yes I am not lazy I want to get better obviously. They treated me like I wasn't even sick. Diet well sodium is supposed to cure everything right or is that just me? They never went into detail on what your so called diet needed to be. Currently for me this is the solution. It goes so much deeper than just a diet. It takes much more.

11.) What medications have you been put on to help with P.O.T.S.? Which ones worked and which ones did not?

Almost all of them in the book. I can't quite remember but I know one suppressed appetite. With this illness and my anorexia. Not a good idea doc. I will eventually put it out on a blog post.

12.) Has the P.O.T.S. disease ever caused you to be depressed or feel like an outcast at any point?

It is beyond horrible in this topic. No matter how much you want to get out.. you can't. You're too sick. So you are alone, depressed only to look at the same walls while talking to yourself. You are exhausted from explaining to others as well. Finding understanding people are hard. I tried to join a support group for lyme disease (none for pots down in FL). They were all too sick to meet up and it got canceled. Blogs have helped me. That and meeting other potsie's online. Vent the app I made some amazing friends and they supported me better than the people around me. Most people did not know I was this ill.

13.) To all those dealing with P.O.T.S. what would be the best advice you could give them to cope with everything that this syndrome entails?

Please don't give up. You still have that fire in you. That anger as well. Use it all. Use all you have and fight this. On the days you cannot do much. Don't let yourself feel bad. We are already dealing with a war. Educate yourself about everything on your illness, on similar illnesses, on the body, the stomach, coping skills for chronic ills, find more inspiration, make new friends online, and create things as much as you can, write about it. Educating myself on every possible possibility was necessary. Even if I wasn't sure I could have something else wrong. Ask for those tests and labs. Because the thing doctors disregarded was that science has questions. You answer a question with a question. It eventually leads to those questions having a answer in themselves. You become more knowledgeable. It is important to be while having this illness. Surround yourself by good things. It is hard to get out so I do recommend the Internet (reviewed and safe). The vent app I used the most. It took time to make the kind of friends and support I wanted on their but it helped me so much. Think about how strong you are. Most importantly think about what you deserve. You deserve love and attention. You deserve to be able to get well again. You deserve to have good people in your life. Don't let this illness tell you no. Don't let those doctors tell you otherwise. The biggest lesson I learned is to stick up for you. Confidence. There are so many inspirational people that were completely outcasted and looked down on. They had to go through hell. Keep fighting because this illness may keep you down physically and mentally. But spiritually it has nothing on you. Do it for the other sick kids and people like you. Keep fighting for them as well. We will tear down POTS one day and those of who did not believe in us. We will fight for what we deserve despite the odds. Another thing that helped me was a chronic playlist I made over time. It is under the user dark wasteland called chronic ill on Spotify.

14.) Do you believe there needs to be more awareness brought worldwide in regards to Postural Orthostatic Tachycardia Syndrome?

There is not enough awareness. Just like anorexia. They ignore that it is major. They still don't teach doctors to know these things. In schools I heard about maybe anorexia once. A chronic illness. Never. I didn't even know what it was until I got one.

Jacqueline, 47 Years Old

1.) First tell me a little bit about yourself? (Name, age, hobbies, anything interesting)

Jacqueline. Age 47. I enjoy photography, and grow my own vegetables. I am unable to work currently. Spent most of my career in restaurant management, on my feet, long hours....doesn't work for me anymore. Am considering filing for disability.

2.) When you were first diagnosed with P.O.T.S.?

Only got diagnosed in 2015.

3.) How long did the process take? How many doctors did you have to see until you finally got an official diagnosis?

I have suffered for 11-12 years, took almost 10 years to get a diagnosis. Truly have lost count of the number of GP's, Cardiologists, Neurologists, ENT"s, Emergency Room visits until a Cardiologist suggested POTS in 2015.

4.) When did you first start noticing something was wrong? First symptom or situation?

Don't remember exactly, do remember being on honeymoon and not able to climb up to an observation deck due to pre-syncope (11 years ago).

5.) Though most causes are unknown do you have any idea what might have triggered the onset of P.O.T.S.?

No, had pneumonia, a tick bite and a Scuba Diving accident (though I feel more confident that POTS CAUSED the accident rather than the other way around) but not sure if any of these caused POTS.

6.) How many trips do you take to a hospital or doctor's office per month? Per year?

Just found an Internist that knows a lot about POTS 2 hours away and have appointments scheduled monthly. I see my cardiologist every 6 months. My new Doc has prescribed Infusions twice weekly. I rarely go to hospital because they don't know what to do for me.

7.) Do you believe you will ever fully recover from P.O.T.S. and never have any setbacks?

I don't believe recovery is an option for me. I just want SOME of my life back! To be able to work, socialize occasionally would be a God send. I don't believe anyone fully recovers.

8.) How has this syndrome affected your work, school, relationships, and friendships? (Life in general)

It has stolen everything from me! I am pretty much housebound, with no outside interests, socializing. It's stolen my personality; I was a social butterfly, happy around people, energized by people. Now, everything zaps my energy. Everything is overload. I worry about passing out in public. Grocery stores are the worst, sensory overload, the lights, the noise, the lines. I feel like my brain cannot process it all. I have lost most of my friends, can't blame them. I bail out of commitments, and even when I'm physically there, I'm not the same person. I'm working through a haze of fatigue, I struggle to find words, any loud noise/light sends me into adrenaline overload. I am not the person that they fell in love with, I smile weekly instead of being the jokester, center of attention cracking jokes, planning crazy weekends. My marriage has suffered. He too has lost the wife he fell in love with. Driven, ambitious, love of life, adventurous, up for anything. I have zero to little interest in physical intimacy, we are now roommates instead of having a loving, close intimate marriage.

9.) What are the worst symptoms you have ever experienced caused by P.O.T.S.?

*Fainting on a guest at the Club I worked at! But I think ongoing is the fatigue and insomnia. Lack of sleep makes my symptoms much **much** worse. And yet, I can't sleep, or stay asleep.*

10.) What has helped you recover the best? (Exercise, food diet, attitude)

Sleep helps. I have been using a recumbent bike regularly since the start of the year. My HR gets up to 175, (leisurely rate), and I feel terrible during and after, but the long-term effects are supposed to be beneficial so I will continue to try. I have put 40lbs on since I became ill, am currently on a weight loss program, which my doctor advised against but I feel it benefits me mentally. On the days that I don't use the bike I aim at my 10,000 steps. Don't often get there, but I like having a goal I can measure myself against. I like to walk on the beach, sometimes I can't, and so I take a chair and sit in a quiet area for an hour. Again, this helps me mentally deal with my condition.

11.) What medications have you been put on to help with P.O.T.S.? Which ones worked and which ones did not?

I was on Florinef .1mg once and then twice per day for 1.5 years. I weaned off because of Edema, and wasn't feeling any benefit.

12.) Has the P.O.T.S. disease ever caused you to be depressed or feel like an outcast at any point?

Yes. No one truly understands. Not even my husband or therapist. They try, but tell me to "buck up", get out there. I truly wish I could. Yes, I believe I'm depressed, I think most people with a chronic illness get depressed. I feel like an outcast because I can't identify with anyone. I can't explain my illness in one word. It's difficult for people to understand, hell, it's difficult for ME to understand lol! If I had cancer, people would get it, if I had a broken leg, people would get it. Invisible illnesses are in some ways harder to deal with, people don't understand. Especially

when, on a good day I can walk 2.5 miles, but on a bad day
I need you to pull right up to the door at CVS!

13.) To all those dealing with P.O.T.S. what would be the best advice you could give them to cope with everything that this syndrome entails?

Rest, listen to your body. Lay down when you can. Salt tabs! Powerade Zero. Join a support group.

14.) Do you believe there needs to be more awareness brought worldwide in regards to Postural Orthostatic Tachycardia Syndrome?

Yes, it's relatively unknown, not studied in medical school. Dr. Grubbs (the Dysautonomia "Guru"), is on a 2 year waitlist! There are a lot of us out there!

Kat, 17 Years Old

1.) First tell me a little bit about yourself? (Name, age, hobbies, anything interesting)

I'm Kat age 17. I love baking, cooking, long boarding and nerd type stuff. Though I don't really get to long board as much anymore since I been diagnosed with POTS

2.) When you were first diagnosed with P.O.T.S.?

2013

3.) How long did the process take? How many doctors did you have to see until you finally got an official diagnosis?

It took about three months. I was admitted 4 times. It was not until I was seen at CHOP (the Children's Hospital of Philadelphia that I got diagnosed with POTS. Dr. Boris diagnosed me right away once he saw me and did something similar to a tilt table test.

4.) When did you first start noticing something was wrong? First symptom or situation?

October 8 2012. I will never forget that day. I woke up and felt terrible with a major headache. I ended up sleeping twenty hours which was not like me at all. Unfortunately, after that, things did not get better they only kept getting worse which lead to me being admitted four times.

5.) Though most causes are unknown do you have any idea what might have triggered the onset of P.O.T.S.?

I was told a combination of mono, puberty, and some traumatic events I experienced when I was younger. The mono really solidified everything I think to trigger the POTS.

6.) How many trips do you take to a hospital or doctor's office per month? Per year?

I have three specialists I see. I see one a month so about 12 times a year not counting the times I may end up in the hospital

7.) Do you believe you will ever fully recover from P.O.T.S. and never have any setbacks?

I was told when I was first diagnosed by different doctors that I had a 50-75 percent chance to outgrow it. Sadly, I do not think that will be the case as I was diagnosed when I was 12 and am now 17. The symptoms have only kept getting worse.

8.) How has this syndrome affected your work, school, relationships, and friendships? (Life in general)

It has affected it tremendously. I have lost friends and do not get out as often as I would like. A lot of my friends do not understand. We will make plans and I will have to end up cancelling them because of how I am feeling. I once had to drop out of school for a little bit of time and be home schooled. My family has tried to understand. They all read a book about POTS but even after they read the book the still have a hard time understanding everything. I have had two boyfriends and neither of the relationships lasted. They would get upset If I did not feel well and was not up to doing something. They could never understand where I was coming from.

9.) What are the worst symptoms you have ever experienced caused by P.O.T.S.?

There are three symptoms that are the worstI experienced. They are headaches, pain and chest pain. The chest pain will get so bad that I end up not being able to breathe and it scares the heck out of me.

10.) What has helped you recover the best? (Exercise, food diet, attitude)

Honestly sleep. Anytime I feel horrible, sleep is what helps me feel better. Maintaining a healthy diet is good too but I would definitely say sleep. I have started acupuncture which has started to make me feel better as well.

11.) What medications have you been put on to help with P.O.T.S.? Which ones worked and which ones did not?

Too many too count. I have been put on several medications that have all caused different side effects. At one point I was on 17 different medications. Right now, I am on 14 different medications. They each help to manage and relieve some type of pain and have been helping so far.

12.) Has the P.O.T.S. disease ever caused you to be depressed or feel like an outcast at any point?

Yes I have suffered from depression. It is hard living in a world where you feel like no one understands you.

13.) To all those dealing with P.O.T.S. what would be the best advice you could give them to cope with everything that this syndrome entails?

Trust me it gets better Keep a positive mind and try to imagine where you will be in 5 years. Do not give up. Believe in yourself and do not let other people bring you down when they tell you it is all in your head.

14.) Do you believe there needs to be more awareness brought worldwide in regards to Postural Orthostatic Tachycardia Syndrome?

Yes, there has been a lot of progress since I have first been diagnosed but it still needs more awareness but the right awareness. People need to be educated. It would be great to be able to explain to someone what you have and for them to know about it and sympathize.

Emily, 21 Years Old

1.) First tell me a little bit about yourself? (Name, age, hobbies, anything interesting)

My name is Emily and I'm 21 years old. I'm interning at a domestic violence center where I use what I've learned being chronically ill to help other people with the things they're dealing with in life.

2.) When you were first diagnosed with P.O.T.S.?

I first became sick in March of 2012 at the age of 16, but wasn't diagnosed until 10 months later in January 2013.

3.) How long did the process take? How many doctors did you have to see until you finally got an official diagnosis?

It took 10 months to get a diagnosis. I saw at least a dozen doctors before one recognized POTS.

4.) When did you first start noticing something was wrong? First symptom or situation?

I went shopping with my mom and we had to come back home because I thought I had the stomach flu. I was nauseous, anxious, tired, and shaky. All the symptoms of the stomach flu. It just never went away.

5.) Though most causes are unknown do you have any idea what might have triggered the onset of P.O.T.S.?

I never had the symptoms of mono, but I had a test that was able to tell me that I was recently infected with the mono virus. So mono is considered to be the trigger of my POTS.

6.) How many trips do you take to a hospital or doctor's office per month? Per year?

For me, it depends. When I'm doing well, I can go months without going to the doctor's office. I've seen 4-5 doctors in a week before when things were bad. For a while, I was getting IV fluids once a month and I still get them occasionally when I feel like I need them.

7.) Do you believe you will ever fully recover from P.O.T.S. and never have any setbacks?

No, I don't think so. I think there will be ups and downs, but I don't think I will ever be completely symptom-free. Even though it didn't start really affecting me until March of 2012, I remember showing minor signs of it, even when I was a little kid. I would get scolded for not picking up my toys because people would think I was lazy, but it was really because it was so uncomfortable for me to bend down numerous times to pick things up off the floor. I thought that everyone felt that way when I was younger, but I've since learned that that's not true.

8.) How has this syndrome affected your work, school, relationships, and friendships? (Life in general)

I was planning on getting my first job the summer after I turned 16, but that's the year I got POTS. I've only just recently been able to handle a part-time internship. I missed many months of high school due to POTS, and multiple days of college classes. I've found that a combination of in-person and online classes is what works best for me. A few months before I developed POTS, I started dating a guy who has stayed by my side through everything. We've been together for over 5 years now. Him and my parents have been my biggest support systems throughout this whole journey. I've gone weeks at a time without seeing him because I was too sick to even have him come over and watch TV. Even though we are still together, it has definitely put a strain on our relationship. We're not really able to go on vacations at this point because of my health, and sometimes I'm not able to keep up with him physically in all of the things we both want to do. Keeping our relationship going in spite of my health has been frustrating and incredibly difficult, but at the end of the day, we both know that we love each other and would do anything to make it work. I've lost many friends because of POTS. A lot of people just don't understand how I can still be sick after all this time and got tired of waiting for me to feel better. Now, it's hard to keep friends because so much of my energy goes into school and work. I have to choose where I spend my energy, and that's what I've been prioritizing the last few years.

9.) What are the worst symptoms you have ever experienced caused by P.O.T.S.?

The nausea and vomiting have probably been the most debilitating. I also have a really hard time sleeping, which contributes to that, as well as the fatigue and headaches.

10.) What has helped you recover the best? (Exercise, food diet, attitude)

Exercise has definitely been the best thing for my recovery. Once I started, it took me quite a few months to notice any big improvement, but I've kept up with it and it has definitely made a difference in how I feel. In order to start exercising seriously, I needed a big attitude change. My life had been completely taken over by POTS, not just physically, but mentally, too. I had to find other things to do and think about, besides dwelling on how sick I felt. I started following fitness accounts on Instagram and doing seated yoga. I bought a bunch of cute workout clothes and would only let myself wear them when I was exercising. This gave me the motivation I needed to turn my mindset around.

11.) What medications have you been put on to help with P.O.T.S.? Which ones worked and which ones did not?

I've tried way too many medications to count. Nausea meds, anxiety meds, beta blockers, etc. They either did nothing or made me feel worse. The only medication that I'm on right now that seems to be helping at all is for hyperthyroidism, which I developed 4 years after I got POTS.

12.) Has the P.O.T.S. disease ever caused you to be depressed or feel like an outcast at any point?

Definitely. It's extremely difficult not being able to do the things that most people my age are doing. I missed out on so much during high school including prom, sporting events, music programs, and social events. That was one of the hardest parts.

13.) To all those dealing with P.O.T.S. what would be the best advice you could give them to cope with everything that this syndrome entails?

Don't let it take over your life. No matter how sick you feel, you have to find other things to do that you enjoy that aren't related to POTS. Even little things, like coloring, yoga, or other hobbies. The more active the better. Push yourself to do things even if you don't feel like it. You know not to push too far, but sometimes you might surprise yourself with the things you can get through. One of my favorite quotes is, "On particularly rough days when I'm sure I can't possibly endure, I like to remind myself that my track record for getting through bad days so far is 100%... and that's pretty good.

14.) Do you believe there needs to be more awareness brought worldwide in regards to Postural Orthostatic Tachycardia Syndrome?

Absolutely. I feel like the lack of awareness for POTS is something that makes life even harder than it needs to be. With more well-known illnesses, people receive support that people with POTS don't get. That can feel very isolating and lonely.

Overall Impression of Stories

These were interviews with numerous questions, but I felt it was important they were all shared. I can relate to a lot of these people since I have the same illness as they do but I hope that even if you do not have P.O.T.S that these interviews had an impact and made you feel some of the ways it made me feel. There was a lot of emotion coming from the interviewees when answering these questions.

As you realize, everyone has a different story, everyone has different symptoms, a different way of getting diagnosed, different medications, and different advice for those dealing with the illness. Two things they all have in common though is feeling the need to bring awareness to P.O.T.S. and that they often get depressed or feel alone and feel as if they will never be cured of the disease. They often feel depressed and alone because to them no one can relate to what they are going through nor wants to understand. Tons of people have never heard of this illness so they do not know what to think. That's why bringing awareness is so important. The more attention that is brought to P.O.T.S and dysautonomia disorders the more educated people can become. The compound effect is the more people that become educated about P.O.T.S.; the people that have P.O.T.S will eventually become less depressed as people will express more understanding and empathy with more education on the illness.

Family Stories

Another interview I conducted was with the family of patients with P.O.T.S. Here you will find interviews with my girlfriend, mother and many other mothers of those with children with P.O.T.S. A lot of times, some family members may not always be honest because at the time they want to protect you. I wanted to get their real thoughts and feelings on how they felt when their child was first diagnosed. I wanted to get their real thoughts and feelings on the process and what it is like to have a loved one suffering from this syndrome. I feel it is imperative people understand not only how it affects the patients but the patients loved ones as well. As you can see this syndrome affects more than just person diagnosed but has a tremendous impact on the whole family. Here are my interviews. Here are their stories.

Here is the nterview with my girlfriend Maddie. At the moment I wrote this, her and I had been dating for a year and 4 months.

1.) What were your first thoughts when I confessed that I had P.O.T.S. and first explained everything to you?

I honestly was not sure what to think. I had never heard of it before. It was really confusing and had no idea what you were talking about. Sometimes it sounded really bad and I was not sure how scared I should be. I have been learning and understanding POTS better as we continue to date and grow together.

2.) What are some difficult things about dating someone who has P.O.T.S.?

This is hard for me to answer because you are such a fighter and always willing to do anything. So if you do

137

not do something I know you are really sick. With that being said that most difficult thing is being scared. There have been numerous times when I have worried about you, when it seems like you are having an attack of some sort. Since you are a fighter sometimes it is difficult because you do things I don't think you should. There have been times when I felt like I should be driving because I can tell you are not feeling very well but you insist on driving anyway"

3.) Do you find it hard to explain to people what P.O.T.S. is when other people ask about your boyfriend's health?"

Yes definitely. It is such a bizarre and complex illness. It is also hard because I do not quite understand it all myself but I am learning.

4.) Have you ever been scared?

I already answered this but yes I have been scared multiple times.

5.) What advice would you give to someone that is dating someone with P.O.T.S.?

Simple. Just listen and try to understand them the best you can. Do your own research.

6.) Should there be more awareness about P.O.T.S.?

Yes it would be great if so many people knew about it and understood it!

Here is the interview with my own Mother:

1.) Did you ever hear about P.O.T.S. before your child was diagnosed?

No

2.) What was your first reaction when you heard your child was diagnosed with P.O.T.S.?

I had no idea what it was. I was shocked because I never heard of it before. So, one of the first things I did was do tons of research to try and learn more.

3.) What scares you the most about having a child with P.O.T.S.? Or if nothing scares you what is the most difficult thing about raising a child with P.O.T.S.?

The scariest thing is the heart issues and that even though there may be nothing physically wrong with the heart it is not comforting knowing that the heart is beating that fast when it does not have to. The most difficult thing is the unpredictability of the syndrome. There are so many symptoms your child has and you never know if it is going to be a good or a bad day for them.

4.) What is one or some of the major differences you have noticed in your child before and after P.O.T.S.?

The biggest difference I could tell is when he would play sports. His athletic motions and strength were not the same. His arms seemed almost weightless and his coordination was not the same as before POTS. It looked as if he was not using all his strength when he really was.

5.) Do you feel there needs to be more awareness to P.O.T.S. and Dysautonomia?

Absolutely. One hundred percent and plus. Even some medical professionals I have spoken with do not even understand what it is.

6.) What advice would you give to other parents that just recently had their child diagnosed with P.O.T.S.?

Do as much research on your own as possible. You will never get as much knowledge as you like in the medical community. Most importantly believe in your child. Trust me at the end of the day your child is not faking it.

Interview with other Mothers:

Story #1

1.) Did you ever hear about P.O.T.S. before your child was diagnosed?

No

2.) What was your first reaction when you heard your child was diagnosed with P.O.T.S.?

I was devastated to be receiving another diagnosis for my children. They were already diagnosed with reflex neurovascular dystrophy, fibromyalgia, multiple allergies, migraines; my oldest also had Lyme disease.

3.) What scares you the most about having a child with P.O.T.S.? Or if nothing scares you what is the most difficult thing about raising a child with P.O.T.S.?

I don't know if I am truly scared but I worry that the kids won't have a satisfying life, careers, relationships, etc. I worry that they will be 100% dependent on me. Not that I mind it, but I want them to be independent and have full lives.

4.) What is one or some of the major differences you have noticed in your child before and after P.O.T.S.?

Before POTS my girls were Irish dancers, they were able to attend school, have friends, be active, make plans,

140

sing, and act in school plays. When they developed POTS they could no longer do the things they loved, especially dancing. They lost many friends; family even stays at a distance. We live moment to moment now. We can't make plans. We spend lots of time at doctor appointments.

5.) Do you feel there needs to be more awareness to P.O.T.S. and Dysautonomia?

Absolutely. Aside from our specialists, most PCP's and ER doctors have no idea what pots and dysautanomia are. I had one doctor tell me that she would get nervous when she saw our names on the schedule. (We only saw her for routine things like strep throat or ear infections)

6.) What advice would you give to other parents that just recently had their child diagnosed with P.O.T.S.?

My advice would be to let go of expectations. Don't compare your child or family life to others. Take each day as it comes and celebrate the positives. Do not dwell on the negatives. Most importantly, always listen to your intuition. You will meet people that will doubt your child. You will meet doctors that will tell you your child is fine. You will meet teachers who think you and your child are making your child's symptoms up. You will be accused of seeking attention. You have to tune it all out and be a fierce advocate for your child.

Story #2

1.) Did you ever hear about P.O.T.S. before your child was diagnosed?

No I had never heard of POTS before my daughter's diagnosis. And the doctor didn't really explain well enough for me to understand. I turned to the internet and oddly Pinterest to find out more.

2.) What was your first reaction when you heard your child was diagnosed with P.O.T.S.?

My initial reaction was shame but thankful we FINALLY had a name for it. For years we would see doctor after doctor with nothing. Checking blood sugar, iron levels, vision and arguing with the school about her attendance. I thought she was a hypochondriac. I mean, her symptoms were all over the place. Every morning stomach ache, later it would be headache, migraines actually, then some random aches and pains. Passing out but a handful of times. Never made any sense to me or any of the doctors we'd see. Then I'd say helplessness was my next reaction/emotion. I feel bad I can't help her enough on her "bad" days.

3.) What scares you the most about having a child with P.O.T.S.? Or if nothing scares you what is the most difficult thing about raising a child with P.O.T.S.?

What concerns me the most is that there is no cure and they treat with medication that has its own side effects that are terrifying.

4.) What is one or some of the major differences you have noticed in your child before and after P.O.T.S.?

I firmly believe she has suffered from POTS since birth or very early on in life, I also feel I have a sister that may have POTS and been wrongly diagnosed.

5.) Do you feel there needs to be more awareness to P.O.T.S. and Dysautonomia?

I definitely think there should be more awareness! During her 4 years of high school I was constantly battling with her attendance, asking if they could help in any way. She was a straight "A" student so they said there wasn't an issue academically but yet they wanted to threaten to fail her or fine me for her attendance. (Wasn't until her junior year we found a doctor that was willing to help and be more involved with the school and truly understood– the first doctor we were seeing, a "POTS specialist", actually told her she was thinking about it too much!)

6.) What advice would you give to other parents that just recently had their child diagnosed with P.O.T.S.?

"Be patient! Your child is not lazy; they are not making this up. Find out a schedule that works for the child. Don't push too hard, one thing I've discovered is that most people that suffer from POTS are extremely hard on themselves and over doers. They strive for excellence, which pushes them too hard for their own bodies.

Story #3

1.) Did you ever hear about P.O.T.S. before your child was diagnosed?

For my older daughter no when my younger daughter was diagnosed we were already a few years in on the oldest diagnoses.

2.) What was your first reaction when you heard your child was diagnosed with P.O.T.S.?

Confusion or relief. Not sure which. I had never heard of it and trying to research it 7 years ago was almost impossible. But I had watched my daughter disintegrate over a period of 8 months or so. I seriously thought she was dying and no one could figure it out. She got sicker and sicker. I had accepted she was going to die. I was just waiting for the doctors to figure it out.

3.) What scares you the most about having a child with P.O.T.S.? Or if nothing scares you what is the most difficult thing about raising a child with P.O.T.S.?

This is going to sound horrible...please understand I am a social worker with a talent for the teen population and I work with many teens. I now have a reputation for being POTS knowledgeable and have worked with a number of families affected by it. My fear would be my girls becoming whiners by my own hand. What I see is 2 types of POTSIES...whiners or warriors. I can see how whiners can easily happen. If my daughter drop something what's the time it's just easier if I bend over and get it for her. There are a lot of adjustments like that that occur when you have children that have issues and I'm sure that's true for any kind of issue. With teens in general they will play most any advantage they are given. It's a hard act to balance. I am in tune enough with my daughters I know when they truly need assistance and I feel they don't try to play that. But the things I have seen befuddles my mind. I am sensitive to POTS and my girls have probably been the worst cases I have come across. The things some of these kids get away with! I would have to make some child abuse reports on myself! Lol! I had one girl who could only wear name brand expensive brands due to the feel of the cheap brands upset her and made her flare...crazy stuff!

4.) What is one or some of the major differences you have noticed in your child before and after P.O.T.S.?

I believe both my daughters are more in tune with their bodies now that they have to make sure they stay regulated. I also feel they have become more empathic since their diagnoses. We all realize that ultimately all of this has a bigger purpose and spreading awareness helps everyone. I also think we as a family are much stronger, resilient, and able to laugh. If we didn't laugh we would always be crying. We have horrified the masses with our reactions to episodes. But ultimately if there isn't an injury it's usually way more traumatic for the spectators.

5.) Do you feel there needs to be more awareness to P.O.T.S. and Dysautonomia?

Yes awareness is so important. I have held quite a few hands on the road to diagnosis. I got lucky. We ended up with a diagnosis before we knew there was 1 issue. We just had back to back illnesses and the gastro seen what was happening and sent us to neuro. Many parents go through not knowing what's wrong not getting any diagnosis.

6.) What advice would you give to other parents that just recently had their child diagnosed with P.O.T.S.?

Stay strong, help your child to be as normal as possible (which means thinking outside the box), know your child better than they know themselves so you know when you can push them or when you should stop them, and all of what I just suggested will take more time and dedication than you would think so be patient.

Story #4

This mother has two kids with P.O.T.S. Here is some background info (Synopsis) before the interview.

Daughter (A) got sick with Cytomegalovirus mid first grade. It hit her like a bad case of mono. (She lost ten pounds, had swollen glands, fever, severe fatigue, etc) The fatigue lessened somewhat, but did not go away. Over the next five and a half years, we saw rheumatology, endocrinology, infectious disease, psychology, neurology, and had a sleep study done. GP thought it was all anxiety and school avoidance. Each year she would start at public school (where she wanted to be). We would 'run out of sick days' and get our bad attendance letter. No diagnosis means no IEP or 504. I have a master's degree in education...I would pull her out of school and homeschool the remainder of the year using the district's curriculum. At the start of seventh grade, we met with a cardiologist from Hershey Medical Center who finally gave the POTS diagnosis. At that point, we gave up on the 'try to attend everyday all day'. We homeschooled, which allowed us to homeschool moat subjects, but it still allowed her to go to school for a couple subject and enabled her to participate in. things like dances (when able). Junior and senior years, we did Cyber School. The curriculum was not very good, but it was our best option at that point. She attends a good college. She lives on campus and has made dean's list most semesters. Fall of sophomore year, she had to medically withdraw. She has taken summer classes to help compensate for the lost semester. She is currently a second semester senior. Sadly she is having a bad flare and we are hoping she does not lose another semester. She is 22. Son (M) became ill two years after A's diagnosis. His diagnosis was much faster because we 'knew the signs', knew to try a poor man's tilt, and had an excellent doctor to advise us. Despite a rough senior year, he was accepted to Bucknell. He has earned excellent grades, but has had to drop out on med withdrawal twice (once for depression and once when having big trouble with hypovolemia). He finished his classwork in December, has a CLEP to do in the next couple months, and will graduate in May. This is a basic synopsis.

1.) Did you ever hear about P.O.T.S. before your child was diagnosed?

Had not heard of POTS before my daughter's diagnosis.

2.) What was your first reaction when you heard your child was diagnosed with P.O.T.S.?

First reaction to the dx (after being told for 5 1/2 years that it was all in her head and that I was just her enabler) was relief that we had a dx and hope that we might have some meds/research/help/emotional support of some sort. When M was suddenly ill and dx, the reaction was more of, "Damn, not again!

3.) What scares you the most about having a child with P.O.T.S.? Or if nothing scares you what is the most difficult thing about raising a child with P.O.T.S.?

Scared? Well...of course there are the concerns of are they going to get through college and then be able to hold down a full time job, etc. Difficult? Hmmm....where to start. It is difficult to keep an eye on meds... Whether they are being taken at the correct time, whether they are the correct dosage, whether they are the correct med (beta blockers cause depression in my kids), etc. Am I taking them to the doctor who is best fit for them? Watching their youth not be what it should. Daughter became the 'empty chair' at school. Kids were nice to her when she was around...but...out of sight/out of mind....she would be overlooked when get togethers occurred. When she did see friends, it would be awkward in groups because she didn't have those unifying experiences of band, sports, dance, shared teachers, etc. Her college experience has been better. M has somewhat the reverse. His childhood included more of the norm in regard to relationships with peers. College experiences were much fewer due to POTS and the fact that he had commuted. Thank goodness for his high school friends who have been loyal and kept in touch.

4.) What is one or some of the major differences you have noticed in your child before and after P.O.T.S.?

POTS had caused brain fog and major fatigue in both A and M. They are both highly intelligent and soon to graduate from great schools. They are both more mature and more empathetic than many peers. The changes I see .... I guess they have had their self-esteem challenged far too often. There are times they are unsure of getting through tasks. But...in many circumstances... I see them stand their ground with grit and determination. They know that it may take longer, but it will work out. Essentially, you cannot direct the wind, but you can adjust the sails. We have learned to let go of things that don't matter.

Back to 3) parenting....It is sometimes very difficult to know when encourage and push....and when to sympathize and protect. Sometimes it is a very fine line.

5.) Do you feel there needs to be more awareness to P.O.T.S. and Dysautonomia?

Yes...awareness needs to happen. doctors need more education about dysautonomia. The public needs more awareness...not only about dysautonomia, but also about other invisible illnesses.

6.) What advice would you give to other parents that just recently had their child diagnosed with P.O.T.S.?

Believe in your child. Advocate for your child. Read up. Educate yourself...don't rely solely on the doctor Join supportive/informative groups such as "POTSibilities.

Parents." Have your child interact in a supportive group...DYNA for younger kids.

Story #5

1.) Did you ever hear about P.O.T.S. before your child was diagnosed?

Yes. Someone shared an article with me after hearing of her symptoms. It was an exact match.

2.) What was your first reaction when you heard your child was diagnosed with P.O.T.S.?

I was confused on how it would affect her but most of all I was sad.

3.) What scares you the most about having a child with P.O.T.S.? Or if nothing scares you what is the most difficult thing about raising a child with P.O.T.S.?

That it will disable her.

4.) What is one or some of the major differences you have noticed in your child before and after P.O.T.S.?

Her quality of life sucks. Things she could do before she can't do now. Her life is forever changed.

5.) Do you feel there needs to be more awareness to P.O.T.S. and Dysautonomia?

Absolutely.

6.) What advice would you give to other parents that just recently had their child diagnosed with P.O.T.S.?

Never let them give up. Fight for them.

Story #6

1.) Did you ever hear about P.O.T.S. before your child was diagnosed?

No.

2.) What was your first reaction when you heard your child was diagnosed with P.O.T.S.?

Our son was 15 when diagnosed. As with others, we had no idea what was happening with our child. When we finally found a doctor who could put a label on what we were dealing with I was so relieved. I thought, if we know what this is, we can start down the path to recovery. It was our first visit to this doctor. He was a neurologist. He said he thought our son had POTS, handed me a sheet of paper from Dyautonomia International told us to set up a follow up appointment with his PA (never got to see this doctor again) and that was it. He did not explain POTS to us at all. He put our son on Florinef and had him continue taking amitriptyline (prescribed by a PED neurologist to try cutting the headaches and dizziness) The doctor told us the push fluids.

I had a meeting at work I needed to get back to, so I put the information sheet on POTS in my purse, dropped my son off at home and went to my meeting. After the meeting, I got back to my office and pulled out the information. I was devastated. I cried so hard after googling POTS. I read about kids who could not stand long enough to take a shower. I read there was no cure, etc. His diagnosis was in Sept 2015. To this day, I am so sad that he has to deal with this.

3.) What scares you the most about having a child with P.O.T.S.? Or if nothing scares you what is the most difficult thing about raising a child with P.O.T.S.?

My son is a strong person and he assures me he would never hurt himself, but that is what I worry about the most. I am worried it will be hard for him to keep his "will to live" when he is sick ALL THE TIME.

I feel terrible that he is sick all the time. He is pale, has insomnia, has lost so much weight, he has stomach issues, head, muscles, etc. Before getting sick he was invincible. It is a lot to take and really hard to not know when the suffering will end. He had to give up a lot. He is so far behind in school that it seems like it will be impossible for him to catch up. His brain fog and concentration has gotten so bad that he can spend a couple hours studying and not remember any of it the next day."

For me, I look at how much he has lost and it has changed the way I parent him. I am fiercely protective and I let him get by with things I never would have before he got sick. For example, when he is feeling better, he wants to be with his friends, but he has TONS of past due assignments. I let him go with his friends. I think, he can take extra time to graduate, if necessary. Ultimately this could be a problem. I cannot decide how hard I should push. My gut says he will know when it is time for him to push himself. First he needs to figure out what he is pushing himself toward.

4.) What is one or some of the major differences you have noticed in your child before and after P.O.T.S.?

Before POTS, my son was very active. Now he is exhausted all the time. He does fairly well in the evenings, but he can hardly function in the mornings. He is on an adjusted school schedule that does not start until 11:00 a.m. but typically he does not make it to school until 2:00. He is so far behind that he is always overwhelmed with makeup work. Before he got sick he hardly ever even had homework.

Also, his disposition has changed. I completely understand but it is hard to see that switch from the life of a carefree teen to the life of a person with a chronic illness. He gets angry when I make appointments for him.He does not have any certainty of when he will feel well enough to go to an appointment.

5.) Do you feel there needs to be more awareness to P.O.T.S. and Dysautonomia?

Yes. I am amazed how many people think this is a psychological illness. Also, when my son is down, he is down. People see him when he is doing better.So, people do not know how much he struggles. We have not had a good morning since he got sick. We have had to deal with people judging him without really understanding what he has.

6.) What advice would you give to other parents that just recently had their child diagnosed with P.O.T.S.?

Join POTSIbilities Parents on FB. Do not count on google searches to learn about this illness. Talk to people who are dealing with it. I just found the POTS support group for parents within the last few months. I wish I had known about it sooner. We were one of the fortunate ones to get a week long appointment at Mayo. Even though I searched for information and read up on POTS, I would have been much better off getting advice on what to ask, etc. from these other parents.

I would tell parents not to pull their kid out of life. The initial information I read said he was exercise intolerant. He was a very active athlete and I pulled him out of football because of my fear. I did learn enough by the time basketball started, so he did play basketball. He does better during basketball season than the rest of the year.

Trust that your child knows their own body. Give them time to grieve, or be angry, etc. Do not push them to "catch back up" Put things in to perspective. In life, we need balance.

Overall Impression of Stories

Just as with the interviews with those currently diagnosed with P.O.T.S., you can tell every mothers story was different. Two things that almost every mothers story had in common was they never heard of P.O.T.S. before their child was diagnosed and the need to bring awareness. Unfortunately, not every child has parents that are as understanding as the ones interviewed, as you may have been able to tell by some of the stories told by those diagnosed with P.O.T.S. I hope with more awareness brought to P.O.T.S. and more mothers like these helping to bring attention to the matter, it will help other parents who have children with P.O.T.S., that are struggling to adapt to their child having this syndrome.

Doctor Interviews

I have dealt with many doctors since I was diagnosed at seventeen-years-old. I wanted to go back and interview some of the doctors that cared for me, as well as ones I heard were specialists in P.O.T.S. The point of these interviews was to see what other professionals thought about P.O.T.S. To those who do not have P.O.T.S. this may help give insight by hearing answer from doctors. At last, I wanted to know what they have experienced firsthand and what may have changed since I was first diagnosed almost a decade ago.

My first interview was with Dr. Jeffrey Boris at the highly regarded Children's Hospital of Philadelphia (CHOP). I was very excited to be able to interview Dr. Jeffrey Boris a P.O.T.S. specialist. He might not be known as well Dr. Blair Grubb out in University of Toledo but the current wait is two years to see him so it was very hard to get an interview. With that said Dr. Boris is easily the second most well-known P.O.T.S. guru in the world and for him willingly to be interviewed for my book was an honor. Here is my interview with Dr. Boris.

1.) Have you ever heard of P.O.T.S.? If so, when and how did you hear about it?

Yes--had remembered seeing something about it in the medical literature back in 2002 when I had a dizzy patient who was not acting like a typical dizzy patient.

2.) Have you ever diagnosed or worked with a patient with P.O.T.S.? If so, approximately how many?

We have diagnosed and cared for over 750 patients with POTS.

3.) There has been a recent increase in people diagnosed with P.O.T.S. Do you have any idea why this might be?

Short answer--no. Long answer--may be better recognition, but may also be some infectious or autoimmune agent.

4.) To the best of your knowledge is it possible to fully recover? Is it possible to ever find a cure?

Yes, but not everyone, and it is not predictable. To find a cure, we must first understand why it happens, which we don't yet. We're working on it.

5.) Do you feel there needs to be more awareness brought to Dysautonomia and Postural Orthostatic Tachycardia Syndrome?

Yes--many doctors have not heard of it. Many others don't believe it exists, and blame the patient (anxiety, conversion disorder, stress) or the parents.

Next was an interview with Nichole Savka. She is currently a nurse and has POTS. She was nice enough to have me interview her from a nurse's perspective.

1.) What do you do as your current profession?

I work as a wound care nurse.

2.) Have you ever heard of P.O.T.S.? If so, when and how did you hear about it?

Before being diagnosed I knew nothing about POTS.

3.) Have you ever diagnosed or worked with a patient with P.O.T.S.? If so, approximately how many?
No

4.) There has been a recent increase in people diagnosed with P.O.T.S. Do you have any idea why this might be?

Possibly chemicals or doctor not looking further into a cause.

5.) To the best of your knowledge is it possible to fully recover? Is it possible to ever find a cure?

I believe people can go into remission. I don't think there will be a cure only because there are so many other diseases that affect the brain and they have not found a cure.

6.) Do you feel there needs to be more awareness brought to Dysautnomia and Postural Orthostatic Tachycardia Syndrome?

Yes I do because people do not understand it and many think it's in your head. Doctors and nurses won't understand it if they haven't heard of it.

Next is Dr. Prathap. A doctor I was able to connect with via Web Md. He is a medicine specialist and has dealt with POTS patients.

1.) What do you do as your current profession?

I am internal medicine specialist.

2.) Have you ever heard of P.O.T.S.? If so, when and how did you hear about it?

I have heard of it.

3.) Have you ever diagnosed or worked with a patient with P.O.T.S.? If so, approximately how many?

I have dealt with several cases. Approximately around 20-25.

4.) There has been a recent increase in people diagnosed with P.O.T.S. Do you have any idea why this might be?

This is being researched at the current moment.

5.) To the best of your knowledge is it possible to fully recover? Is it possible to ever find a cure?

It's not always possible to have full recovery, it depends on the insight the patient had in his/her condition and the adherence to preventive measures.

6.) Do you feel there needs to be more awareness brought to Dysautonomia and Postural Orthostatic Tachycardia Syndrome?

It needs to be recognized in society. People need to be educated about the preventive measures and treatment of POTS.

Next is Dr. Shinas Hussain who I was also able to connect with via Web Md. He also has an experience with a POTS patient.

1.) What do you do as your current profession?

I'm working as a medical officer under National Health Mission (NHM)

2.) Have you ever heard of P.O.T.S.? If so, when and how did you hear about it?

Yes, I have seen a case in my training period and there was a discussion about POTS.

3.) Have you ever diagnosed or worked with a patient with P.O.T.S.? If so, approximately how many?

As I said I met with a patient during my internship. I have seen only one case of POTS in my career.

4.) There has been a recent increase in people diagnosed with P.O.T.S. Do you have any idea why this might be?

In the past, POTS cases were under reported. It is a diagnosis of exclusion. Due to advanced diagnostic tests and increased number of hospital visit among general population more and more cases are reported. I'm of the opinion that the number of cases remains the same but reported cases increases.

5.) To the best of your knowledge is it possible to fully recover? Is it possible to ever find a cure?

According to my knowledge prognosis is good. Most of the people recover with prompt pharmacological therapy and life style modification, but treatment may be needed for many years.

6.) Do you feel there needs to be more awareness brought to Dysautonomia and Postural Orthostatic Tachycardia Syndrome?

Definitely. More awareness is needed both for patients and physicians.

Next is an interview with the guy who is my cardiologist. He is Dr. Russo at Berks Cardiologist. He is one of the best cardiologists I have had and am glad he was able to help me out with an interview.

1.) Have you ever heard of P.O.T.S.? If so, when and how did you hear about it?

Yes, in medical school.

2.) Have you ever diagnosed or worked with a patient with P.O.T.S.? If so, approximately how many?

Yes I have. I have worked anywhere with between 5-10 patients.

3.) There has been a recent increase in people diagnosed with P.O.T.S. Do you have any idea why this might be?

More awareness among doctors. Better non-invasive and heart tests. This leads to more diagnosis of POTS.

4.) To the best of your knowledge is it possible to fully recover? Is it possible to ever find a cure?

To my knowledge it is not possible to fully recover and no cure. There are treatments for symptoms.

6.) Do you feel there needs to be more awareness brought to Dysautonomia and Postural Orthostatic Tachycardia Syndrome?

Yes, because it can be a very debilitating disorder.

Overall Impression of Stories

I wish I could have done more interviews but I realized it is very hard to get an interview with a doctor. Doctors have a very important role and are very busy. Also, being a first time author many may not have wanted to take the time out for an interview or did not want to do something that did not involve getting paid. I am not sure why but trust me I tried. I made numerous phone calls, sent out several emails as well as delivered a good number of personalized notes. I did have several doctors respond saying they do not know much about the illness and did not feel qualified to interview, which as you can see by even the remarks made by P.O.T.S. guru Dr. Boris, is that there is even quite of bit doctors that never heard about P.O.T.S. This is quite alarming, considering the fact it was discovered in 1993 and been around for over twenty years. What is more concerning is there have already been one million people diagnosed, but imagine how much higher that number might be if every doctor was aware of this disease. My final remarks on the doctors interviews are, again, every doctor's experience is different but they all have one thing in common. They all agree we need to bring more **AWARENESS.**

My Research

For this book I decided to do an amount of research on my own, as you will see later in my questions and illustrations in this chapter. With successful marketing through multiple social media outlets I had over 2,000 people participate on the survey, I conducted through survey monkey, which for illustration and better comprehension purposes I convert in to percentages of 100. Previously, I have told my own story, interviewed several other P.O.T.S. patients and; family members as well as medical professionals knowledgeable of the diagnosis.

With this survey, I want to give the general perception of what the average people in today's society know and feel about P.O.T.S. I wanted to see how many were aware of the disease. How they felt about it or if they felt they needed to know more. I wanted to see if there was a certain judgement or bias towards P.O.T.S. patients or if the issue was just simply a lack of knowledge.

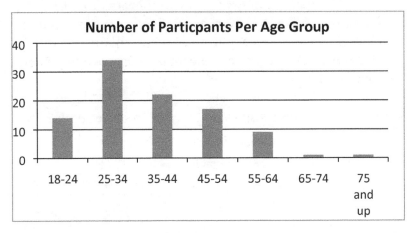

As you can see I sampled from a good wide variety of age groups for my survey. Fourteen percent were between the ages of 18-24, thirty-four percent were between the ages of 25-34, twenty-two percent were between the ages of 35-44, seventeen percent between ages of 45-54, nine percent between ages of 55-64, three percent were between the ages of 65-74, and even one percent of people above the age of 75. More women than men participated in the study.

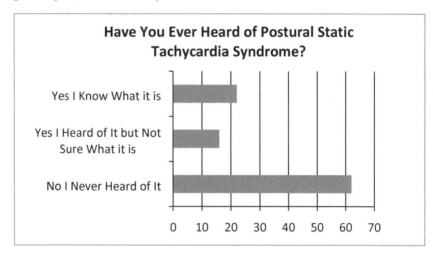

For the question, had they ever heard of P.O.T.S.? Not surprising, over sixty percent of people never heard of it before. Sixteen percent heard of it but still did not know what it was. Only eighteen percent of people actually knew what P.O.T.S. was.

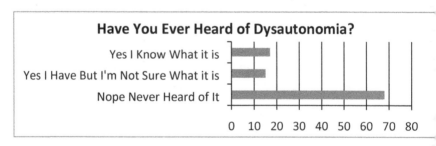

Results were very similar when asking if they ever heard of dysautonomia, which is the type of disorder

P.O.T.S. is. Again, over sixty percent never heard of it. Fifteen percent heard of it but did not know it was, and only seventeen percent of people actually knew what it was.

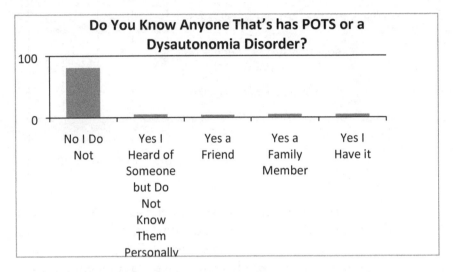

As illustrated above eighty percent of people do not know anyone that currently has P.O.T.S. or a dysautonomia disorder. Five percent heard of someone but did not know them personally. Five percent actually had the illness and ten percent knew a family or friend that was diagnosed.

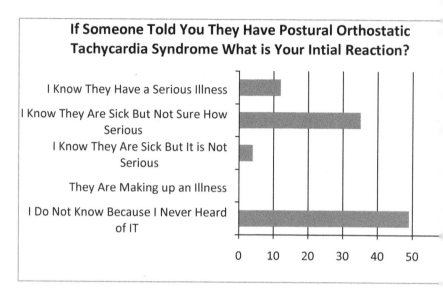

If Someone Told You They Have Postural Orthostatic Tachycardia Syndrome What is Your Intial Reaction?

This question I was very interested in. As you heard from most people, they feel judged when they tell someone they have P.O.T.S. So, I wanted to ask the general public what their reaction would be if someone told them they had P.O.T.S. Almost half the people responded that they do not know how they would act because they never heard of it. Thirty-five percent stated they would know the person was sick but not sure how serious it was. Twelve percent said they knew it was a serious illness, meanwhile four percent said they thought it was not serious. An encouraging sign was that not one single person believed they were making up an illness.

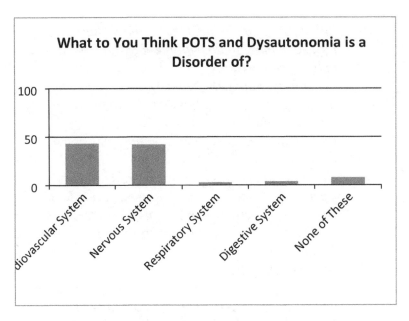

What to You Think POTS and Dysautonomia is a Disorder of?

When I asked what people thought P.O.T.S. was a disorder of; most people were split between the cardiovascular and nervous system. Forty-three percent said cardiovascular and forty-two percent said the nervous system. Eight percent though it was either the respiratory or digestive system while another eight percent believed it was none of these.

Last but not least, I wanted people to comment on even if they had no idea what P.O.T.S. was if they had to give an educated guess what they thought it might be. I got a wide variety of answers. Some were spot on, while some were very surprising. Here are the answers.

Please Give a Brief Statement is to what you feel Postural Orthostatic Tachycardia Syndrome is Whether You Heard of It or Not?

➢ *I think Tachycardia has to do with heart rhythm. But other than that I have no idea.*

> *Still learning, my daughter may have this and may have something to do with the fact that she had multiple concussions.*

> *Something to do with the heart.*

> *I'm going to assume it has something to do with the blood flow due to the name.*

> *A psychological condition affecting the central nervous system.*

> *I can only guess based on some prefixes and root words "post" and "ortho" to assume it has to do with being "correct position", making me guess something isn't upright or functioning the way it should.*

> *Autoimmune disease*

> *POTS is an insidious thief of quality of life. Each movement of sufferers must be calculated to determine safety, necessity, risk, and benefit. POTS robs people of normalcy, employability, and often a sense of self.*

> *I think it's a lump or pain in the back of your head.*

> *Something to do with your spine?*

> *I've never heard of it. But now am curious about it."*

> *Never heard of it*

> *Based on just the words, sounds like something related to a rapid heart rate depending on which position your body is in. However I have no idea!*

> *I remember looking up POTS on google once. However, that's all I really remember. I believe it related to seizures.*

> *A debilitating disease that's very difficult to treat. It often makes simple parts of life unbearable. Standing, staying hydrated, temperature changes, physical activity, etc.*

> *Something with the back*

> *We have had a number of students diagnosed with POTS in recent years. I know they have to watch*

their diet and salt intake. I had one student wear a
patch behind his ear because it helped with the
symptoms. I *think* it's an autoimmune disease and
there are a variety of symptoms. No known cause
though some people blame vaccines (possibly
cervadil/vaccines for HPV).
> *Some kind of disorder of the bones.*
> *I have heard of POTS before but only in reference. I*
  never learned what it was.
> *Valves of the heart aren't functioning properly*

After doing all this research I realized a couple things.
It has been repeated a bunch of times but first and foremost
is the need to bring awareness and educate. More than half
the people had no idea what P.O.T.S. or dysautonomia was.
Even more surprising was with currently one million
people being diagnosed worldwide was that eighty percent
never knew anyone that was diagnosed. The answer for this
is simple and one I can relate to very well. Most people
diagnosed with P.O.T.S. do not want to tell anyone. Since
no one is aware or educated, people can come off as they
do not understand, they do not believe you, or they do not
know what to think. If everyone that had P.O.T.S. was not
afraid to tell anyone that answer would have been a lot
higher.

The most positive thing to come out of this survey was
that a lot of people seem very interested. I had people reach
out to me, exclaiming after my survey they started googling
and were intrigued to learn more. Another positive was that
not one single person believed it was a fake illness. As
someone with P.O.T.S., I found this hard to believe but this
could be contributed to a bunch of factors. They could have
researched during that question possibly or they do not
want to come off arrogant since they were not sure if the
survey may have been anonymous or not. Another reason is
when something is being heavily researched they know it is

not a fictitious thing. Last but not least, what I take from this is that when people seem to not understand when someone with P.O.T.S. tells them they have P.O.T.S., it has nothing to do with they do not believe you or they think you are making it up. As humans we have natural emotions and sometimes let those get in the way and make quick assumptions like that. The reality is most people do not have the proper education when it comes to P.O.T.S., so in all honesty do not know how to react. They believe you; they just want more schooling on the issue.

My New Outlook

After a week went by and lots of deep hard thinking I accepted to leave my position as assistant branch manager with the Hertz Corporation. It seemed as if Postural Orthostatic Tachycardia Syndrome was something that you never completely get over and can flare up at any given time or moment. I always dreamed of being self-employed and running my own business but I was too scared to take the risk. I also kept convincing myself that it was never the right time. After everything I had just been through, my gut was telling me that now might be the correct time. I had my doubts if I could ever work for someone else. I did not trust that my health would be able to live up to my employers' expectation. Continuing down the path of being an employer just seemed like it would end up being a never-ending cycle. I would recover from P.O.T.S. get a new job, make a good impression and work my way up only to a couple years later have to leave or be fired due to something that triggered a relapse to my P.O.T.S. syndrome. I am twenty-five years old, fortunate to live with dad and not have to pay rent. I also do not have any current children.

At the same time, I was only getting older and those circumstances will eventually end up changing before I know it. It was time to stop being scared and just go for it. I had my business degree. Business was something I was always good at. I won the "Most outstanding Student in Business Award" my senior year of high school. I needed a career that could let me work on my own hours and pace. This may be the only way I could sustain success having P.O.T.S. If I wanted to be successful it looked as if being a business owner or self-employed was the answer.

When I was still working at Hertz I made a decision to work part-time for Primerica Financial Services. I got my life insurance license with the state of Pennsylvania. In my spare time, I could sit down with families, coach them on their finances and possibly make extra income. I loved Primerica and everything the company stood for. It gave me the opportunity to start and create my own business. I would have loved to leave Hertz and done it full-time sooner but again I was scared because living on commission was not guaranteed income. I felt I needed to save up before I made this choice. Besides going full-time in Primerica, I also started up my own limited liability company "DEVS LLC". It was a music marketing, songwriting, and mentor company to help out inspiring musicians in the area. Ever since I was younger I wrote music. I loved to write songs, mostly hip-hop and R and B. It was my second passion behind sports. I decided to try and make my passion a reality. This business is something I have started doing and trying to build up on the side as well as Primerica. Along with these two businesses as you all know I decided to write this book and started writing articles for SB Nation. I could no longer play sports but that did not no longer mean I could not write about them.

Being self-employed is daunting because everything falls on you. With that being said, being self-employed and being your own business owner has so many positives. I love having the ability to work when I want to and having the freedom to create my own schedule. I can tell my attitude and happiness have all increased because of this.

My outlook on health has changed since all this started. I no longer believe I will ever fully recover with no setbacks. This is going to be a battle I will have to fight my whole life. I however, refuse to let this battle defeat me. It can be intimidating but the mindset I decided to adapt was if anything bad happens, I rather have it happen with me trying to live my life to the fullest the best I can than to have it happen with me just laying around wasting time and living life with anxiety.

With everything that has happened to me in my past I now know it is imperative that I take extremely good care of my body. Maintaining a healthy diet, having a constant exercise plan is so much more important to me than the average Joe. The same goes with being sure to limit my alcohol and caffeine intake. For my diet, I have limited myself to only fast food and desert once a week. I do not drink any soda or caffeine. I drink water, Gatorade, milk, protein shakes, and lemonade. That is it. I follow a strict exercise plan. Every Monday, Wednesday and Saturday I go for one short walk in morning and light weight lifting at night. On Tuesday and Wednesday I go for short walk in the morning and another at night. These are to keep my strength and cardio levels maintained well. I start out very light. My goal is to eventually increase that I can start running and jogging again. The end goal is to start swimming. An exercise I enjoy more than running. I have already seen progress in the past month I have started implementing this new work out plan.

I have not had any alcohol since I had my last relapse which has now been over five months. A part of me does not want to drink ever again. With that being said I am a typical guy and I love to have a beer or two during a football game or at the bar with the fellas. Until my P.O.T.S. improves, any alcohol is not an option right now. Once my health is better I may have a beer or two during a game once in a blue moon but it is imperative it is only once in a while for the outlook of my future health. I feel this is not just for me but significant for anyone living with P.O.T.S.

Last but not least, I started seeing a reflexologist. My mom had a friend who started up her own reflexology clinic and I decided to give it a try. To be honest it has worked wonders. It is amazing how many points in our feet connect with other parts of our body. I truly believe medicine is not the best way to go. In my experience it seems like more beneficial for the pharmaceutical business than anything else. This is why they make it so difficult to wean of certain drugs. Yoga, acupuncture and reflexology are great natural options for the body and things I would highly recommend. I did yoga in college and reflexology currently. They both make me feel better, reflexology exceptionally so.

As mentioned before, I mentally accepted the fact I will never ever recover from P.O.T.S. No doubt this is discouraging but it has seemed to increase my motivation. I have dreams and I refuse to let this syndrome take my dreams away from me. This type of motivation is not so easy to always maintain especially when you have an illness that drains so much energy out of you. To keep my motivation level and spirits high I have started listening to motivational speaker podcasts, playlist, and songs on my morning walk. Continuing to work on self-improvement has helped me tremendously in my battle with P.O.T.S. Listening to these audios usually gets me in the proper mindset to take on the day and fight through whatever symptoms I may encounter throughout the day. I seem to appreciate life more to. Life is hard. P.O.T.S. makes life really hard physically at times. Everyone has struggles. I realize I am not the only person that life is hard for. Everyone person no matter race, gender, income level is battling something we do not know about. In this world full of negativity, I want to have a positive outlook and hopefully start to spread that to others. Besides my best friend dying a young age, P.O.T.S. has also taught me that anyone's life can flash right in front of their eyes at any moment so let's enjoy every one minute we get of it. We have to start spreading awareness to all things that need to be recognized. This is one of the reasons that I decided to write this book.

My Advice to Those with P.O.T.S.

Unfortunately, I have dealt with P.OT.S. the past eight years. I have been through many doctors and plenty of trips to the emergency room. Starting my senior year of high school, I went through college and started an everyday entry level career battling this ugly syndrome. I have quite the experience and if there is an anything other P.O.T.S. patients are struggling with I would love to help. Regrettably, this syndrome is hard to understand unless you experience it yourself. It is incredibly nice to be able to reach out to those who are going through the same thing as you. To those who have years of experience dealing with a wide range of symptoms or those that have been just recently diagnosed with P.O.T.S. I hope you can easily relate to many things I have talked about from many different levels. You should expect to find this chapter helpful if you are open minded to advice and willing to try some new things to help cope with your symptoms or anything P.O.T.S. may be causing you to go through.

In this chapter I will give you advice on how to deal with this syndrome mentally, physically and emotionally. I will also go over topics such as how to exercise, medications, and from a diet standpoint. Before I start giving some of my advice I want to be clear that I am not a doctor and Postural Orthostatic Tachycardia Syndrome is a very strange syndrome with many symptoms. What may work for others and I may not always work best for you. I still think it never hurts to hear other people's experiences and gather other people's advice. There may be something you have not tried and with a syndrome so new and so much research to be done. I would encourage everyone to never stop learning and to be open minded to trying new methods.

First, I will start with diet. Every doctor encourages increasing your salt intake to try and get the blood flowing throughout your body more efficiently. This may work for some. This never quite totally worked for me. You should increase your salt intake but be careful how you increase it. Increasing it too much or a certain way can have negative consequences. For instance, eating a bunch of fast food would not be the correct way. Drinking plenty of fluids, yes but stay away from soda, especially caffeine. Caffeine will increase the effect of your tachycardia. What worked for me was drinking plenty of fluids. I drank my water and I had a small bottle of Gatorade a day. Maintaining a healthy diet, cutting out fast food and deserts while getting your electrolytes and sodium is what worked best for me. It really is true when people say you feel better when you eat better. This is not different for P.O.T.S. In fact, since dealing with P.O.T.S. you feel worse than the normal person anyway, a proper diet is more important than it would be to an average person. This means eating all three meals a day with little snacks in between. You need food for energy. Be sure not to over eat. Overeating will draw more blood to the stomach and less to your head, hence increasing your P.O.T.S. symptoms. Eat three light meals and if you are hungrier throughout the day, eat little snacks. No matter where you go always make sure to keep a drink on you to stay hydrated. I personally usually carry a water bottle on me at all times.

Next I will talk about exercise. Now as bad you might feel and as fast as your heart may race upon standing up or due to exertion, a little exercise is a must. As long as you can do something without passing out I would encourage doing it. Lying around will only make your symptoms worse. Start out by short walks. Then continue to increase the length of your walks slowly. Light weight lifting will help you as well. Weightlifting makes you feel stronger. Overall, when it comes to exercising the key is balance. Start out slow but make sure you are progressing. If you progress and it makes you feel worse, please slow down, rest and start over again. Eventually, overtime if you keep at this you will see improvement. It is important in life that everyone gets proper exercise. It is especially important for P.O.T.S. patients. Even though you may feel like doing nothing but lying around thinking the rest will make you feel better, you are wrong. If all you do is lay around it can make the symptoms worse to the point you will end up passing out minutes upon standing. If not worse, the symptoms will definitely stay stagnant.

I wish there was some proven medicine that could heal P.O.T.S. but unfortunately there is none at this time. Talk with your doctor and notify him of your worse symptoms. This way they can try and prescribe you something to help lessen those symptoms. If you are having anxiety, which is increasing your symptoms, speak with someone about anxiety medication. If P.O.T.S. has caused you to be extremely depressed, talk to someone about going on an anti-depressant. For me no medication seemed to help my physical symptoms. I am a firm believer in diet and exercise is the key to relieving P.O.T.S. symptoms. Natural things such as massages, yoga, acupuncture and reflexology as previously mentioned have made me feel better as well.

However, with the syndrome I would become extremely depressed at times. I was put on an anti-depressant which worked for me to a point I did not need it anymore. Unfortunately, the mediation was so strong that no matter how hard the doctor tried my body could not wean off it which is my reason for frustration at the pharmaceutical industry. Despite that, the medication did keep me motivated even when I was feeling terrible at my lowest time. Medications are going to be like trial and error. Just continue to work with your doctor until you find the right one.

This leads me to the next part in how to deal with P.O.T.S. from an emotional point of view. P.O.T.S. can take a toll on you. It changes your lifestyle, cause you to feel like an outcast and miss out on many things. You will experience sadness and anger. Anti-depressant meds can help but the medicine will not just work by itself. I was lucky to have loyal friends whom I was very honest with in what was going on with me. They would pick me up all the time. If I needed to sleep in the car they would let me but at least we were out doing stuff. They were people I could talk to for a support system. A support system is imperative to your success emotionally. P.O.T.S. is new and misunderstood by so many people. People may seem to look at you like you are crazy or being lazy. You look fine on the outside but they do not realize what is going on in the inside. This is the curse of an invisible disease. They are unaware you are suffering from a dysautonomia disorder. This is why it is so important to find someone that understands you. It will make you feel ten times better knowing that you have someone to talk to. This can be a parent, relative, friend, husband, wife, brother, sister, girlfriend, or boyfriend. Either way it is significant you are open and honest about your condition. The more people you are open and honest with, the more likely you are to find someone that understands you. In fact, you might also find someone else that has or no someone that also has P.O.T.S. If you absolutely do not have anyone, I would encourage looking for a counselor to talk to. It is important to talk to someone about how you are feeling. Keeping everything inside is not going to help your symptoms. If money is an issue for a counselor, there is a Postural Orthostatic Tachycardia Syndrome group on Facebook. On this group people blog and post about their problems this syndrome has caused them. I would encourage joining this. It will remind you that you are not alone.

Last is the mental aspect. In order to beat P.O.T.S. you are going to have to be mentally tough in order to not have P.O.T.S. beat you. You need to stay upbeat and constantly believe things will get better. You need to wake up every day with the mindset to improve your condition. You cannot just lie around and wait. If you lie around and wait thinking something is magically going to happen to improve how you are feeling, you are wrong. I do not mean for this to come off as tough guy talk (think of it as tough love) but I know this from true personal experience. You might not be able to run, play sports or do all the things you use to all the time. There may be some things you may never be able to do again. This does not mean life is over. There are so many things that you can pursue in life. Research other hobbies that you think you can do and start pursuing them. It is important to stay busy. This will take your mind off things and how you feel at times. This is probably the biggest aspect in living with P.O.T.S. No matter how well you diet, how many people you talk to, what medication you take, how much you try and exercise, if you do not have a positive, motivated mindset and continue to work on self-improvement you are never going to fully live a life you dream of again.

I hope this helps. As stated before everyone is different but I think these are some important things to put in perspective. It is also vital you find a good doctor as well. Not every doctor will know about P.O.T.S. and some will know more than others. It is imperative you find a doctor you feel comfortable with. Once you find this doctor stick with them. This will help speed up the process. It also will give you someone that can continue to monitor you and let you know how you are progressing throughout the years.

Let's Bring Awareness

The other day I was on Facebook when I scrolled across a video one of my Facebook friends shared. The reason the video caught my eye was because by surprise it started out by saying how this person had Postural Orthostatic Tachycardia Syndrome. It was a video about a teenage female with P.O.T.S. and how she trained her dog to help assist her when her P.O.T.S. would get so bad that she could not do the simple things like laundry or load the dishwasher. The video was inspiring and amazing how well the dog was trained and how compassionate the animal was towards her companion suffering from P.O.T.S. Dogs have great instincts and that dog definitely knew its owner was sick, or else the dog would never have been so willing to train and learn all that stuff. Who was not compassionate however was my Facebook friend who decided to share the video with everyone. Instead of commenting on how cool it was to see a dog act the way it did or help spread positive awareness about P.O.T.S, my Facebook friend decided to comment that "Seems like a lazy bitch to me." He was referring to the teenage female who was suffering from P.O.T.S. He believed nothing was wrong with her. He thought the reason this lady trained this dog was so she did not have to do anything. He never understood the full struggle this teenager dealt with on a day in and day out basis.

After seeing this post, I was upset. I wanted to comment and reach out to the person who posted it. I decided not to. I knew arguing on social media never does any good. In fact, it usually does more harm. It did however provide more ambition to write this book and made me realize more than ever how we have to start creating more awareness for this life altering syndrome. Instead of doing more research on the syndrome, by simply googling it, the person made an assumption based on what he saw in the video. This person like many others saw a perfectly looking female teenager, not realizing she had a dysautonomia disorder. He never lived a day in her shoes and never knew how she was actually feeling. This still did not stop him from making an insulting assumption. That person did not realize or know what it feels like to have tachycardia. He did not realize what it is like to have your heart racing up to 160 beats per minute upon standing. This can sometimes be higher or lower depending on the person's level of severity with P.O.T.S. It just goes to show, as quick as everyone is to google something in today's society, the sad reality is you still have a lot of people who will not research before making assumptions

This person's response is why so many people with P.O.T.S. as you can tell by the many that have so willingly shared stories feel like an outcast. Some people can be so quick to judge and no one is willing to listen or learn. The syndrome is really hard to understand. Part of the problem is because it is so new and unknown. With it being new and unknown, there has not been much media or national exposure to it. As my survey has shown me to believe there are more good people than bad in this world. All P.O.T.S. needs is more education and a little worldwide exposure. If more people knew about P.O.T.S., including doctors, things would be a lot different. If I was diagnosed right away instead of going through three months of doctors' visits, consistently being told it just anxiety and in my head, things would have been a lot different. It would have been a lot easier on my family and everyone around me. When no one knows about P.O.T.S., and every doctor is constantly telling you the same thing, most people are going to believe the doctors no matter what you say. Unfortunately, this story is familiar with a lot of P.O.T.S. patients and it needs to change. The only way it can change is with awareness.

It is time we start bringing awareness to P.O.T.S. I will start by doing this myself. The word needs to get out there. Family, friends, coworkers, or anyone that knows anyone that is suffering from P.O.T.S. is going to need to help out as well. Remember big teams accomplish big dreams. More and more people are being diagnosed with this syndrome. The time is now and I am willing to make this happen. There are so many ways to raise awareness now a day's, whether it be through social media, TV, newspaper, or fundraising events. If we all work together we can help the people suffering from P.O.T.S. feel more accepted in society and willing to come out and be open about their illness. We can make them believe they still have a chance to achieve their goals in life. I am not one to ask people for money but if you or you know someone that would ever be interested in raising money for Postural Orthostatic Tachycardia Syndrome you can donate or do a fundraiser for the "Red Lily Foundation". This foundation uses funds to help research hoping to eventually find a cause and cure for P.O.T.S. The website is redlilyfoundation.org.

P.O.T.S. is a dysautonomia disorder. So you can also bring awareness to dysautonomia or fundraising for them would help as well. A good foundation for this is the National Dysautonomia Research Foundation and can be found at www.ndrf.org. If you are reading this book and want to learn more, I encourage you to google and research. You will be surprised at all you will find. You can also YouTube "Postural Orthostatic Tachycardia Syndrome.' Besides videos put out by doctors describing what P.O.T.S. is you will find many people suffering from P.O.T.S. that post their own videos and blogs about how they are suffering. A lot of times these videos are the best because you can actually see for yourself what a P.O.T.S. attack or even a fainting spell upon standing looks like.

Conclusion

Everyone in their life has a story, this is mine. Everyone in life is struggling with something or knows someone that is struggling with an issue that needs awareness brought to light. Mine happens to be Postural Orthostatic Tachycardia Syndrome. Some people know at a young age what they are meant to fight for in the world. They had experiences that happened to them as child that stuck with them as an adult. Others do not realize until they are nearing the end of their life what they want to fight for. At 25, with my experience I realized my fight was going to be to bring awareness to P.O.T.S. and to give back to everyone that has endured what I have if not worse with this illness.

I hope this book can reach out and inspire people. For those that have read this book. I hope you enjoyed this book as much as I enjoyed writing it. Even if you did not enjoy it, the very least I hope you have gained awareness and knowledge of Postural Orthostatic Tachycardia Syndrome. That was the main purpose I decided to write this in the very first place.

If you would have asked me even two years ago if I would ever write a book I would have told you "No way." I never would have imagined in a million years I would write a book and be known as an author. I never had the ambition or desire. I got good grades, mostly A's and B's in school because there was punishment for poor academics. To be honest I never really liked school. I hated typing and writing assignments in high school and research papers in college. It is crazy how as time goes on, things will happen in life and your views start to change. Things we enjoyed when we were younger, we no longer enjoy. Stuff we never thought we do we end up pursuing. This is often because of shift in mindset as we get older, as we mature and experience different things. Sometimes it can be due to life circumstances.

After having my last setback with P.O.T.S. at twenty-five years old I decided it was time to be honest with everyone. It was time to bring awareness. I knew one way would be to write a book. I knew it would be a lot of work but something in my gut was telling me it would be worth it. I questioned if I could be motivated enough or physically able to do it but once I started typing it was like I could not stop; mind over matter. It is amazing how much you can write when you are just telling a true life story of things that have happened to you that you are so passionate about. I was no longer just typing BS to fill up space on a research paper. Everything flowed. As this began to happen, I became more and more confident I was making the right decision. When all the people started supporting me and helping me out with interviews this was just the icing on the cake. I saw the support I was getting and knew I could not turn back. I realized people were starting to put faith in me. I gave them hope when often they felt hopeless or like no one understood them. There was no way I was going to let them down. This leads me to my last part.

I would like to thank all the people that have helped me put this book together, read this book, and encouraged me in the process. First, I would like to thank all the interviewees that are currently suffering from P.O.T.S. for participating in the interview. You were such a big help in not only this book but as we all continue together to fight for awareness and more medical answers. I was amazed at how different but yet very similar are experiences were. Some were better, some worse than others but we all had one thing in common which was P.O.T.S. We also all have the desire to continue to educate not only ourselves but others about this terrible syndrome. I had never written a book before and for you to be able to trust me in making this book happen means a lot.

Next, I like to thank all the doctors who have worked with me ever since my diagnosis with P.O.T.S. I have seen so many and you each played a part to get me where I am today. The doctors that took their time out to be interviewed, your help was tremendously appreciated. You are all so busy and I am blessed that you would take your time out to help me with this.

Last but not least I want to thank my mom (Lisa Morganti), dad (Chad Evans), step dad (David Morganti), brother (Kyle Morganti), sister (Sarah Morganti), and all my family and friends. You all have supported me so much during my hard times and always kept me going when I did not feel like it. There were so many times that you all sacrificed a lot just so you can tend to me when P.O.T.S. had me at my weakest points. For those who know me I am a man of few words but do not think that a day goes by that I do realize what you all have done. I love you all and together we will all bring awareness.

We will bring awareness to Postural Orthostatic Tachycardia Syndrome (P.O.T.S.), a dysautonomia disorder, a syndrome that has so many symptoms, a syndrome that changed and affected so many lives, a syndrome that has taken lives due to suicide and a syndrome so new, with so little known about it. It is a syndrome with no yet known cause or cure, a syndrome that can be so life altering and debilitating, and a syndrome that is so hard to understand and comprehend. It is such a rare syndrome, one that can show your vital signs as if and make you feel like you are physically so close to dying......, yet only to be told you were actually so far away.

About the Author

Derek Chad Evans was born and raised in Reading, Pennsylvania where he currently resides to this day. Derek was born Easter Sunday March 31, 1991 to Lisa Morganti and Chad Evans. Growing up, as early as five years old, when he first started playing youth soccer, Derek found his love for sports. He often dreamed of playing professionally.

He always loved helping others and has volunteered and hosted many charity events. At seventeen-years-old he was diagnosed with Postural Orthostatic Tachycardia Syndrome which meant his dreams of professional sports would no longer be a possibility. Derek graduated high school from Exeter Township in 2009. During his senior year, he won the Most Outstanding Student in Business Award. He later attended Indiana University of Pennsylvania (IUP). He graduated in 2014 with a Major in Sports Administration and a minor in Business Management.

He worked at the Hertz Corporation in his home town coming out of college, where he worked his way up to Assistant Manager. Derek had to resign from Hertz due to a recent setback in his P.O.T.S. in early October 2016. This was one of the biggest factors in encouraging him to write this book. Derek has recently gotten back on his feet, starting up his own business DEVS LLC and working as a financial advisor for Primerica Financial Services. He also enjoys writing articles for SB Nation. To learn more, you can follow Derek on Twitter, Instagram, and Snapchat @DerekCEvans, or on Facebook at Derek Evans.

Glossary

A

ADHD: a chronic condition marked by persistent inattention, hyperactivity, and sometimes impulsivity. **ADHD** begins in childhood and often lasts into adulthood. As many as 2 out of every 3 children with **ADHD** continue to have symptoms as adults.

Alopecia Areata: a type of hair loss that occurs when your immune system accidentally attacks hair follicles, which is where hair growth begins. The damage to the follicle is usually not permanent.

Anoxic Seizure: seizures that occur after an area of the brain suffers a drop in oxygenation due most often to a lack or decrease in blood supply. These are very different than epileptic in origin, and are most often found in the very young.

C

Chronic Fatigue Syndrome/CFS/ME: systemic illness marked by > 6 months of fatigue, and over 8 more symptoms and signs. ME is Myalgic Encephalomyelitis and is another name for the illness.

Conversion Disorder: a mental condition in which a person has some neurologic complaint such as blindness, paralysis, etc. that cannot be explained by medical evaluation.

D

Dysautonomia Disorder: a term for a group of diseases that include postural orthostatic tachycardia syndrome (POTS), multiple system atrophy, autonomic failure, and autonomic neuropathy. In these conditions the autonomic nervous system (ANS) does not work properly.

E

Eczema: a medical condition in which patches of skin become rough and inflamed, with blisters that cause itching and bleeding, sometimes resulting from a reaction to irritation (eczematous dermatitis) but more typically having no obvious external cause.

Edema: is the abnormal accumulation of fluid in certain tissues within the body. The accumulation of fluid may be under the skin - usually in dependent areas such as the legs (peripheral **edema**, or ankle **edema**), or it may accumulate in the lungs (pulmonary **edema**).

Ehlers Danlos: a group of genetic connective tissue disorders. ... EDS is caused by a defect in the structure, production, or processing of collagen or proteins that interact with collagen. The collagen in connective tissue helps tissues resist deformation.

Electrocardiogram (ECG/EKG): the process of recording the electrical activity of the heart over a period of time using electrodes placed on the skin.

Endorphins: any of a group of hormones secreted within the brain and nervous system and having a number of physiological functions. They are peptides that activate the body's opiate receptors, causing an analgesic effect

G

Gait: a person's manner of walking.

Ganglion Cyst: a fluid-filled noncancerous lump that usually develops in the wrist or hand. But some occur in the ankles or feet. When a **ganglion cyst** presses on a nerve it can be painful. And depending on its location, a **ganglion cyst** may restrict movement.

I

Infarction: the obstruction of the blood supply to an organ or region of tissue, typically by a thrombus or embolus, causing local death of the tissue

Intravenous Immunoglobulin (IVIG): A sterile solution of concentrated antibodies extracted from healthy people that is administered directly into a vein. Abbreviated **IVIG**. IVIG is used to treat disorders of the immune system or to boost the immune response to serious illness. Also, known as **intravenous** gamma globulin (IGG).

M

Mastocytosis: a disorder that can occur in both children and adults. It is caused by the presence of too many mast cells in your body. You can find mast cells in skin, lymph nodes, internal organs (such as the liver and spleen) and the linings of the lung, stomach, and intestine.

Myalgic Encephalomyelitis: abbreviated as ME, is one of several alternate names for the disease that's commonly known as chronic fatigue syndrome (CFS). ... The word **myalgic** means muscle pain or tenderness. my is a shortened form of myo, which means muscle.

P

POTS= **Postural:** Pertaining to the posture or position of the body, the attitude or carriage of the body as

> a whole, or the position of the limbs (the arms and legs). **Postural** hypotension is a drop in blood pressure (hypotension) due to a change in body position (a change in posture).
>
> **Orthostatic:** relating to or caused by an upright posture
>
> **Tachycardia:** a common type of heart rhythm disorder (arrhythmia) in which the heart beats faster than normal while at rest.
>
> **Syndrome:** a group of symptoms that consistently occur together or a condition characterized by a set of associated symptoms.

Potsies: People with POTS

Premature Ventricular Contraction (PVC): are extra, abnormal heartbeats that begin in one of your heart's two lower pumping chambers (ventricles). These extra beats disrupt your regular heart rhythm, sometimes causing you to feel a flip-flop or skipped beat in your chest.

Presyncope: a state of lightheadedness, muscular weakness, blurred vision, and feeling faint (as opposed to syncope, which is actually fainting). **Presyncope** is most often cardiovascular in cause. ... In many people, lightheadedness is a symptom of orthostatic hypotension.

Proprioception: The unconscious perception of movement and spatial orientation arising from stimuli within the body itself. In humans, these stimuli are detected by nerves within the body itself, as well as by the semicircular canals of the inner ear.

R

Rheumatoid Arthritis: a chronic progressive disease causing inflammation in the joints and resulting in painful deformity and immobility, especially in the fingers, wrists, feet, and ankles.

S

Scoliosis: abnormal lateral curvature of the spine.

T

Tilt Table Test (TTT): occasionally called upright tilt testing, is a medical procedure often used to diagnose dysautonomia or syncope.

U

Urticaria: a rash of round, red welts on the skin that itch intensely, sometimes with dangerous swelling, caused by an allergic reaction, typically to specific foods.

V

Ventricular Septal Defect: a defect in the ventricular septum, the wall dividing the left and right ventricles of the heart. The extent of the opening may vary from pin size to complete absence of the **ventricular septum**, creating one common **ventricle**

References

1.) "Dysautonomia International: Postural Orthostatic Tachycardia Syndrome." *Dysautonomia International: Postural Orthostatic Tachycardia Syndrome.* Dysautonomia International, 2012. Web. 19 Mar. 2017.

2.) "Postural Orthostatic Tachycardia Syndrome." *National Institutes of Health.* U.S. Department of Health and Human Services, May 2016. Web. 19 Mar. 2017.

3.) "Postural Orthostatic Tachycardia Syndrome (POTS) - Topic Overview." *WebMD.* WebMD, 2017. Web. 19 Mar. 2017

4.) "Stand Up!" *Red Lily Foundation.* Red Lily Foundation, 2017. Web. 19 Mar. 2017.

5.) "Home." *Dysautonomia Advocacy Foundation.* Dysautonomia Advocacy Foundation, 2017. Web. 19 Mar. 2017.

6.) "Blair P. Grubb, MD." *Blair P. Grubb, MD.* University of Toledo, 2017. Web. 19 Mar. 2017.

7.) Evans, Derek C. *SurveyMonkey-POTS and Dysautonomia.* Survey Monkey, 22 Feb. 2017. Web. 19 Mar. 2017.

8.) "Tilt-Table Test." *Tilt-Table Test.* American Heart Organization, 2017. Web. 19 Mar. 2017.

9.) "NDRF." *NDRF.* National Dysautonomia Research Foundation, 2017. Web. 20 Mar. 2017.